# Praise for Jorge Cruise

"Jorge Cruise takes a three-pronged approach to weight loss and overall health."
—*Harper's BAAZAR*

"Lose weight without cutting out your favorite food groups."
—*REDBOOK*

"This challenge helped me get past years-long plateau—I haven't been this skinny since high school."
—*Allure*

"Cruise offers a flab-melting, low stress diet."
—*Life & Style*

"Jorge Cruise guarantees we're going to be looking beautiful in that bathing suit."
—*CNN*

"Jorge, again, is on to something; belly fat is surely an indicator of poor health."
—Suzanne Somers, #1 New York Times bestselling author of *Ageless: The Naked Truth About Bioidentical Hormones*

"Jorge Cruise has answers that really work and take almost no time. I highly recommend them."
—Andrew Weil, bestselling author of *8 Weeks to Optimum Health*

"I'm eternally grateful to Jorge for creating a simple lifestyle plan."
—Christiane Northrup, M.D., #1 New York Times bestselling author of *The Wisdom of Menopause*

"Jorge knows what he's talking about. Follow his book—lose the weight."
—*Chris Robinson, fitness expert and author of* The Core Connection

"Jorge Cruise will keep you looking and feeling your best."
—David Kirsch, author of *The Ultimate New York Body Plan*

"Jorge continues to inspire and make losing weight fun and part of your life forever."
—Mariel Hemingway, author of **Healthy Living from the Inside Out**

"Sets you up to win!"
—Anthony Robbins, bestselling author

tiny
and full™

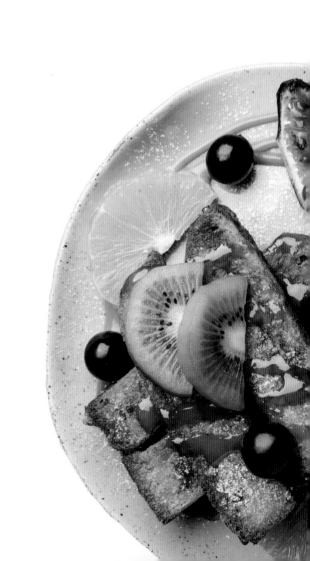

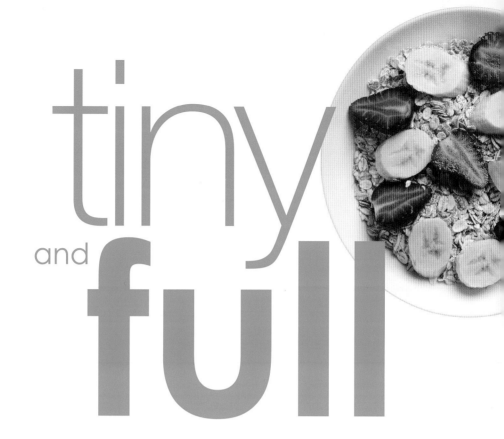

# tiny
## and full

Discover Why Only Eating a
Vegan Breakfast Will Keep
You Tiny and Full for Life

## Jorge Cruise

BENBELLA BOOKS, INC.

DALLAS, TX

Trademarks:

| | | |
|---|---|---|
| Tiny and Full™ | Wake Up Vegan™ | Jorge Cruise™ |
| 8 Minutes in the Morning™ | 3-Hour Diet™ | Belly Fat Cure™ |
| Carb Swap System™ | The 100™ | Sugar Calories™ |
| Happy Hormones, Slim Belly™ | Women's Carb Cycling™ | Skinny Waffle™ |
| Stubborn Fat Gone!™ | Move Fit™ | |

BenBella Books, Inc.
10300 N. Central Expressway
Suite #530
Dallas, TX 75231
www.benbellabooks.com
Send feedback to feedback@benbellabooks.com

Printed in the United States of America
10 9 8 7 6 5 4 3 2 1

Library of Congress Cataloging-in-Publication Data is available.
ISBN-13: 978-1-942952-48-0

Editing by Heather Butterfield
Copyediting by Karen Levy, Julie McNamee,
 and Eryn Carlson

Proofreading by Jessika Rieck and Brittney Martinez
Printed by Versa Press, Inc.

Distributed by Perseus Distribution
www.perseusdistribution.com
To place orders through Perseus Distribution:
Tel: (800) 343-4499
Fax: (800) 351-5073
E-mail: orderentry@perseusbooks.com

**Significant discounts for bulk sales are available. Please contact Glenn Yeffeth at glenn@benbellabooks.com or call (214) 750-3628.**

To my fiancé, Sam,

For making coming home

always the best part

of my day.

# Contents

# Foreword

I recently enjoyed a delightful dinner in NYC with my dear friend of over a decade, Jorge Cruise. We caught up about one another's lives and families, of course, but then devoted much of our time together to a discussion of Jorge's new book—this book—*Tiny and Full*. I have since had the opportunity to read the book, and here are a few impressions.

Jorge has always had, and continues to have, a unique ability to take complicated information and make it simple and accessible. In particular, I consider him genuinely gifted when it comes to seeing an easy way into an important healthy behavior change that most people find intimidating. That is certainly the case with *tiny and full,* which addresses the many good reasons for eating more plant-based diets that many of us talk about all the time. But then, in that inimitable Jorge Cruise style, the book serves up a brilliantly simple insight that never dawned on the rest of us: go vegan in the morning! Suddenly, what might have seemed an imposing burden of change is bite-size, and manageable. Suddenly, you can get there from here—and then, perhaps, keep going.

As a physician focused on disease prevention and health promotion, Jorge knows that "tiny," the use of which he explains, is his choice but not mine. While he is quite right about waist circumference as a potent indicator of metabolic health, and the waist to hip ratio in women an indicator of reproductive health that has had implications for attractiveness and sex appeal throughout history and across all cultures, you certainly don't need to be "tiny" to be healthy, and my focus is health and vitality. If we take the liberty of interpreting "tiny" to mean a healthy waist circumference, then we are aligned. It's not about size; it's about vitality.

I particularly appreciate how Jorge combines insights about motivation, behavior change science, and the benefits of plant-based eating to offer the empowering simplicity of this plan. Frankly, I like how it conforms to my personal experience as well. I am a very disciplined person, fully committed to practicing what I preach. Even so, I find it much easier to practice that discipline, and get my workouts in, in the morning. At the end of a long and challenging day, I like to kick back and relax like everyone else.

The focus of my career, including the newly launched *True Health Initiative,* is all about leveraging the incredible, and all-too-often neglected, power of lifestyle as medicine. The centerpiece of a health promoting lifestyle is a diet of wholesome foods, mostly plants, in sensible combinations.The clever and innovative guidance in that direction served in *tiny and full* is moderate and manageable, encouraging and inviting. My hope is that you accept the invitation to join Jorge for breakfast, and step in the direction of the true, vibrant beauty that only health and vitality confer.

**David L. Katz, MD, MPH, FACPM, FACP** is the founding director (1998) of Yale University's Yale-Griffin Prevention Research Center, and current President of the American College of Lifestyle Medicine.

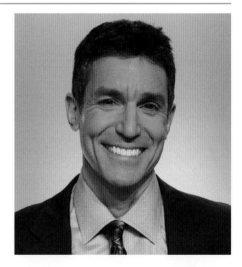

He earned his BA degree from Dartmouth College (1984); his MD from the Albert Einstein College of Medicine (1988); and his MPH from the Yale University School of Public Health (1993). He completed sequential residency training in Internal Medicine, and Preventive Medicine/Public Health. He is a two-time diplomate of the American Board of Internal Medicine, and a board-certified specialist in Preventive Medicine/Public Health. He has received two Honorary Doctorates.

Dr. Katz has published roughly 200 scientific articles and textbook chapters, and 15 books to date, including multiple editions of leading textbooks in both Preventive Medicine, and nutrition. He has made important contributions in the areas of lifestyle interventions for health promotion; nutrient profiling; behavior modification; holistic care; and evidence-based medicine. A widely supported nominee for the position of U.S. Surgeon General, Dr. Katz has been recognized by Greatist.com as one of the 100 most influential people in health and fitness in the world for the past 3 years (2013-). He is recognized globally for expertise in nutrition, weight management and the prevention of chronic disease, and has a social media following of well over half a million. He has delivered addresses in numerous countries on four continents, and has been acclaimed by colleagues as the "poet laureate" of health promotion. In 2015, Dr. Katz established the True Health Initiative to help convert what we know about lifestyle as medicine into what we do about it, in the service of adding years to lives and life to years around the globe.

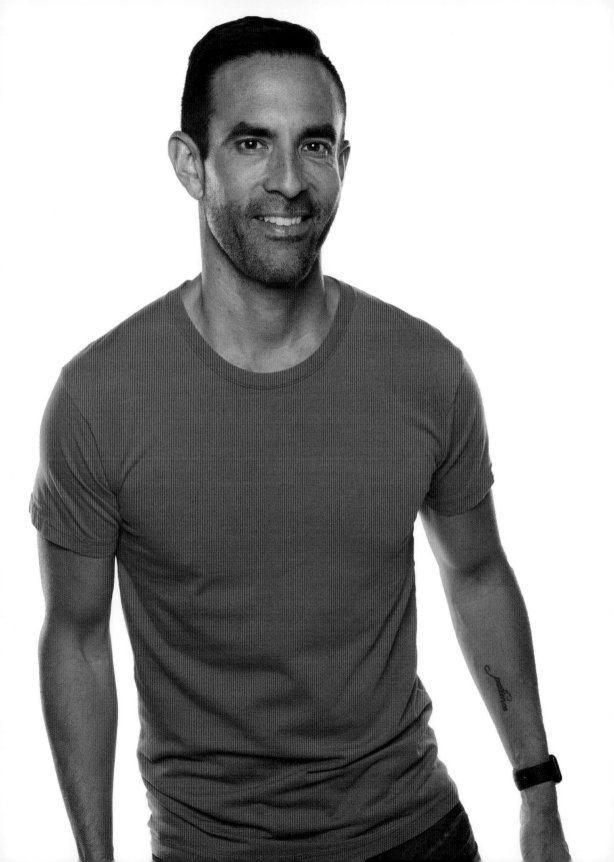

# Welcome

*From the desk of Jorge Cruise*

Dear Friends,

**What if I told you that your breakfast holds the power to total health, natural weight loss, and increased all-day energy?**

Well it's true! I am so thrilled that you are here and that I have the opportunity to share this message with you. I have been a celebrity fitness trainer for the past 15 years, and it has all come down to this lifestyle plan that will work far beyond the 12 weeks described in this book. I want to welcome you to the Tiny and Full™ revolution!

**So what's it all about? Waking Up Vegan!**

The vegan diet is more popular than ever, and people all over the world are touting its healthful benefits—longevity, energy, and even weight loss. For most of us, though, it's a lifestyle change that is just too hard to maintain. More important, it's missing crucial nutrients for optimal wellness.

With *Tiny and Full*™, you only have to Wake Up Vegan™ to see the results of a plant-based diet. You'll discover that eating vegan at just one meal—breakfast—is better for you than if you ate vegan all day long. This plan is about more than just weight loss. It's about epic health! If you are currently a vegan, this message may seem alarming to you and you may be ready to put this book down, but I encourage you to read on and give me a chance to change your mind.

I've also given you a straightforward meal plan and an energetic fitness program, plus 50 of my most mouthwatering, delicious recipes—from a Tropical Mango Blast smoothie and Grilled Tilapia Grapefruit Salad to a Tomato Gazpacho Fresca and even Banana Berry Ice Cream. I will guide you every step of the way for 12 weeks, over which you should expect to lose one to two pounds every single week. You will soon be on your way to confidence, vitality, and health!

This book provides all the guidelines you need to transform your body and improve your life—starting now! I am so glad you're here!

Happy reading!

Your Coach,

*Jorge Cruise*

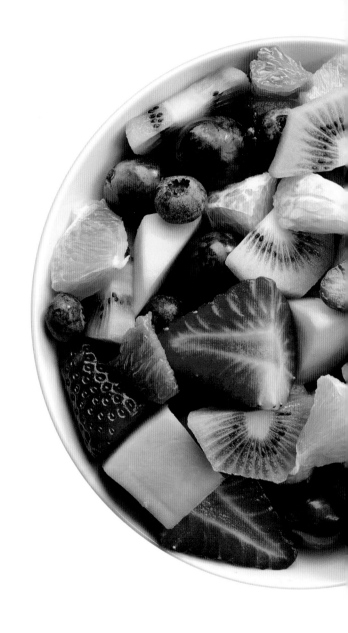

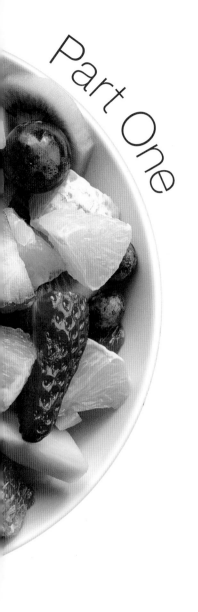

# The
# Wake Up
# Vegan™
# Revolution

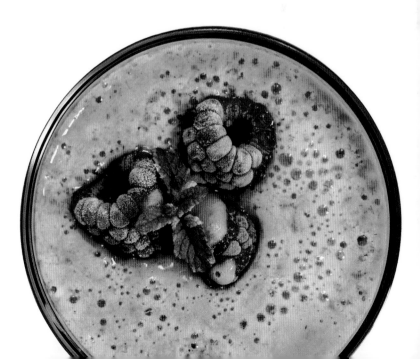

# 1 Ready for Tiny

3

Getting "Ready for Tiny" means many things. First and foremost, you must understand that *Tiny* is a frame of mind. It's a shift from thinking that you have to settle for *some* weight loss and a *little* less flab to owning that you not only have the power to be perfectly Tiny, you deserve nothing less. Yes, you have the right to be Tiny!

## What exactly is Tiny?

Tiny isn't about vanity or some narcissistic need to stand in front of the mirror obsessing about being the fairest of them all. It's the understanding that you have the absolute inherent power and right to be as red-carpet gorgeous, fit, and healthy as any celebrity beauty. Tiny doesn't have an age limit, and it isn't just about looks—being Tiny *is* about being healthy. In fact, far from being fanatical, Tiny is actually *the* number one indicator of health and fitness—having a Tiny Waist *is* epic health, inside and out. *Your outside beauty indicates your inside health.*

Did you get that? Both things, inner beauty and outer beauty, are inherently related. Looking and feeling good on the outside—fitting effortlessly in your skinny jeans, being a showstopper in your little black dress, rocking a bikini—is a reflection of your inner health. That's what having a Tiny Waist gives you: outer beauty and inner health. The great reality is that having a Tiny Waist is a reliable gauge of underlying whole-body wellness, vitality, and health. With this knowledge, you can and *should* embrace being beautiful, without fear of being labeled egotistical or superficial. A small waist gives you beauty, energy, and confidence; attracts other people to you; *and* lowers your risk for all diseases. We'll get into this in great detail on the next pages, but for now, know that having a healthy waist circumference—having a Tiny Waist—frees you to be the best *you* ever. When you harness this powerful mind-set—the mind-set of Tiny—you are Ready for Tiny.

Now . . .

Are *you* Ready for Tiny?

First, we must address three points:

1. How a Tiny Waist equals health

2. How to get a Tiny Waist

3. How to beat THE problem: hunger!

After we've covered these points, you'll be ready to commit to your health for the next 12 weeks—to promise yourself that you will get a Tiny Waist, which will free you to be the best *you* ever. You'll be free to wear that bikini with joy and free to never diet again.

Let's start by taking a deeper look at how slimming your middle will give you an overall body and mind health makeover.

## A Tiny Waist Equals Health

In 2009, I had the great privilege of sitting down with Dr. Mehmet Oz for an interview. I'll never forget that day. Despite an incredibly busy schedule of filming his own show, Dr. Oz had invited me and my team to film a short video for my readers while he was on a layover in New York. That day I learned some vital distinctions about waist circumference that I'd never before considered. I came away from our talk with a thrilling new insight—that wanting, no, *needing* a slender waist truly isn't about vanity but is instead an essential requirement for true health and fitness.

Your waist circumference, Dr. Oz told me, simple as it seems, is a key marker of health, vitality, disease, happiness, risk of heart disease, stroke, and many cancers. It's also the main attraction, or detraction, when choosing partners—and not for the trivial reasons you might suspect.

According to the research of Devendra Singh, an evolutionary psychologist at the University of Texas who published the pioneering findings on the significance of attractiveness and waist size, first impressions are belly-based. Singh's research on waist-to-hip ratio spans 1993 through 2010, just before he passed away. He was the first to reveal the link between having a Tiny Waist and attractiveness and health. One such study found that attractiveness is gauged by waist circumference—with thin being in and fat being out. Singh's paper reviewed three separate studies, which all concluded that men define the attractiveness of women based on their low waist-to-hip ratio (more on waist-to-hip ratio on page 7):

- The first study had men rate the attractiveness of pageant contestants over the past 30 to 60 years. The raters consistently decided that the tinier the waist, the more attractive the women.

- The second study concluded that college-age men find women with small waists more attractive, healthier, and of greater value as reproductive partners than women with thicker waists.

- In the final study, men aged 25 to 85 were found to prefer women with smaller waists and rated them as being more attractive and having a higher fertility rate.

What does this mean? Six-pack sizzle and the hotness factor aside, these men are not making superficial choices. Singh concluded that these preferences for slim waists are actually linked to health. These men were really being attracted to health. It's easy to think that the unrealistic photoshopped pictures of beauty that we often see promoted in the media are what sway men to choose slim-waisted women, but, in reality, women with Tiny Waists *are* healthier. In a jointly published study from a prominent university in Spain and the University of Wisconsin, researchers found that higher amounts of belly fat in women are linked to increased risks for ovarian disease and infertility. Even more shocking, according to a study published in the *Journal of the American Medical Association*, increased waist size is consistently linked to increased risks of cardiovascular disorders, adult-onset diabetes, elevated plasma lipids, hypertension, cancer (endometrial, ovarian, and breast), gall bladder disease, and premature mortality in women. So this fondness for Tiny-Waisted women is really a natural tendency to select a healthier partner.

And men aren't the only ones "sizing up" their potential mates—women find slim-waisted men more attractive as well. In a study published in the *Journal of*

*Personality and Social Psychology,* two experiments were conducted to examine how women choose mates:

- In the first group, college-age women rated normal weight male figures with lean and thick waists. The women consistently rated males with leaner waists as being more attractive and healthy and as containing more positive qualities than the men with thicker waists.

- Women ages 18 to 69 rated men with a variety of waist sizes. All women, regardless of their age, education, or income, rated men with the leanest waists more favorably than those with thicker middles.

And the links to waist size and health in men are just as evident as they are in women. Studies done by researchers in Texas, Australia, and Sweden connected high levels of belly fat in men directly to low levels of available testosterone. These researchers speculate that high levels of abdominal fat on a man convert testosterone to estrogen, which lowers sperm count and causes lack of muscle. Experts who study mate choice and attractiveness speculate that the trend for choosing mates based on Tiny Waists comes from our evolutionary history. This preference for Tiny Waists, researchers believe, is in fact a deeply ingrained evolutionary adaptation that dates back more than 160,000 years.

According to researchers who study ancient humans, it seems that our ancestors instinctively knew to avoid mates with large bellies because they were an indicator of poor health. These ancient humans didn't have the constant stream of 24/7 media telling them how to choose a mate. They had to go by instinct to tell them which man or woman would make the best partner in terms of provider, protector, and reproductive partner. So, the idea of "sizing someone up" may have had its start back among prehistoric humans. Besides doing a general once-over for a healthy body size and shape, it turns out that belly size is an easy to spot and reliable indicator of a high-quality or poor-quality mate. As for Paleolithic women, the researchers speculate that they had a biological instinct not to choose a big-bellied caveman because he wouldn't be a strong protector, efficient provider, or good reproductive partner. On the flip side, if a Paleolithic man saw a woman with a large belly, researchers think his instinct would alert him that she was either pregnant (and therefore unavailable) or might have a hormonal imbalance such as ovarian disease, which could decrease her ability to reproduce.

The bottom line is that regardless if you are male or female, a high waist circumference is a marker of serious health issues, and "a hot body is an instinctual sign of health," as Dr. Oz so beautifully states in his book, *YOU: Being Beautiful: The Owner's Manual to Inner and Outer Beauty.*

So, stop feeling guilty about wanting a Tiny Waist. It's hard wired. Accept that having outer beauty is a reflection of inner health. This is your new mind-set. You aren't shallow, vapid, or vain—you want a Tiny Waist because you want optimal health. Looking smoking hot is just something you'll have to live with.

## What is a Tiny Waist?

Your waist-to-hip ratio is the measurement that best shows how Tiny—or not—your waist is. Figuring it out only requires a fabric tape measure, you, and some very simple math. Take a tape measure, and while sucking your belly in, measure your waist at the level of your belly button. Next, measure your hips at the largest point around your bottom. Finally, divide your waist size by your hip size. An ideal ratio is 0.8 for women and 0.95 for men. Canadian researchers said that this test is an ideal and inexpensive way to predict something as serious as heart disease.

If your waist circumference is higher than these results, don't fret. This book is designed to help you lose one to two pounds a week over the course of 12 weeks. *Tiny and Full*™ will give you long-lasting, sustainable results. You'll get the body you want, and it will stay the body you dreamed of forever.

# Waist to Hip Ratio

| Female | Male | Related Health Risk |
|---|---|---|
| .80 or below | .95 or below | Low |
| .81 to .85 | .96 to 1.0 | Moderate |
| .85 or higher | 1.0 or higher | High |

# How to Get a Tiny Waist

You have to cut calories. Period.

There.

I said it.

I didn't come to this conclusion easily, folks. I've been a calorie-bashing, fruit-banishing, nut-noshing, spinach-with-chicken-salad–eating enthusiast for years now. I have published books, posted blogs, and tweeted regularly and passionately about only "counting the calories that count" or, worse, "not counting calories at all." But, calories are the key to weight loss, and I've finally seen the light.

Whatever the diet, this is the new reality—you must create a calorie deficit if you want to shed pounds, lose belly fat, and get a Tiny Waist. Now I know that this isn't really "new," but for some time now, the most popular diets, from Atkins to South Beach, The Paleo Solution to The Primal Blueprint, and, yes, The Belly Fat Cure™ to The 100™ (those two are mine), all promise weight loss without tracking or counting calories, or at least not all calories. To be fair, many of these plans do (and my diets also do) provide menus that are low calorie, so they do result in weight loss (as long as the reader follows the menu to the letter). The faulty premise of most of these diets is the claim that you'll naturally eat less because you'll be eating more filling and slowly digestible foods, and also that you won't be eating foods (refined sugars and flours that spike insulin) that cause fat accumulation. Unfortunately, these claims don't hold. The first idea—that you'll naturally eat less—doesn't hold because most of us don't stop eating just because we feel full. Many physical, emotional, and psychological reasons regulate how much food we consume and when we stop eating. Brian Wansink, professor of consumer behavior at Cornell and author of *Mindless Eating,* has conducted several clever studies that repeatedly show that the more food you put in front of you, the more you eat. It doesn't matter what it is—we humans always eat more than we should. We are simply lousy at randomly limiting ourselves to an appropriate amount of calories. Second, while avoiding refined sugars and flours is still a good rule of thumb, if you *don't* cut overall calories, you *won't* see weight loss. There is no one food component that causes fat accumulation, as some fat enthusiasts argue. Finally, diets that focus on cutting out an entire food group—all fruits and grains, for example—are too severe and are unsustainable even when they do cut calories. The result is that most people eventually go off these plans and binge on the forbidden foods.

The idea of fat accumulation as being the result of insulin-spiking foods (all carbs and sugars) is one that I once wholeheartedly endorsed, but in the light of more recent and accurate studies, I now reject this theory. I was one of many who loved the message of Gary Taubes, an engaging and gifted journalist, who has written many books and articles that claim carbohydrates are solely responsible for obesity and fat accumulation. Taubes argues that it's impossible to lose weight while eating carbohydrates, but that you can achieve weight loss by eating as many calories as you desire as long as you cut out all carbs and sugars. This all boils down to the way that insulin, says Taubes, spiked by carbohydrate-rich foods, causes fat to be accumulated. The research does not bear out, however. More recent and careful studies provide evidence which shows that more calories, regardless of type, means more weight, and vice versa.

In 2015, a new National Institutes of Health study published in *Cell Metabolism* examined the effects of low-carb and low-fat calorie-controlled diets on 19 obese men and women. The participants stayed in a metabolic unit for two weeks so the

## Cutting Calories Any Way You Please

When it comes to weight loss, it really doesn't matter how you slice away the excess calories—reduce your intake and you'll drop the pounds. There are no promises of great health here and I don't recommend any of the following diets, but when it comes to moving the needle on the scale down, cutting calories is the key. The following outrageous examples illustrate just how crazy diets can be:

- **Twinkies:** To show that all calories—even the emptiest—count, an overweight Kansas State University nutrition professor put himself on a self-professed Twinkie Diet on which he ate one of the Hostess treats every three hours and interspersed the Twinkies with snacks of Doritos chips, sugary cereals, and Oreos. He limited himself to roughly less than 1,800 calories a day of the overly processed, highly refined, sugar-and-fat-filled diet and lost 27 pounds over the course of 10 weeks. The professor to date hasn't released any health issues resulting from his diet.

- **Baby Food:** Yes, this Hollywood fad of substituting baby food for two, or possibly three, meals a day does result in weight loss. Celebrity trainer Tracy Anderson started this gimmick for cutting calories and controlling portions, and although it does cause weight loss (as long as you are cutting your calories), most people who tried it reported that the weight quickly returned when they started eating adult food again. This diet is an Internet phenomenon and isn't published anywhere, but it makes sense when you use baby food, which is around 20 to 100 calories per jar, to replace a meal that would typically be 300 to 500 calories.

researchers could control, regulate, and record all food intake and activity. Each group cut their daily calorie intake by 30 percent. Half of the group cut carbs (low carb), and the other half cut fat (high carb). After the two weeks, the subjects took a break for a few weeks, and then they came back and repeated the study, with the two groups switching diets. Interestingly, the average participant lost about a pound of fat over two weeks and about four pounds of weight, but the high carb group lost *more* body fat (the high-carb group lost 463 grams of fat on average, compared to 245 grams in the low-carb dieters). Further, the researchers predicted that had the diets continued over the following six months, the people in the high-carb group would have ended the study losing six more pounds than the low-carb group. This directly debunks the popular low-carb theory purported by Taubes which claims that low-carb diets are more effective for fat loss because they lower levels of insulin and therefore liberate fat from fat tissue. This dispels the theory that only low-carb diets can help people shed fat. The bottom line is, once again, overall calories matter most for weight loss. (For more on my philosophical transformation, see page 11.)

For the record, I still believe that refined sugars and flours and overly processed foods cause serious health issues, but they aren't the reason for weight gain or loss—that's all about calories. You can just as easily lose weight eating 1,200 calories of Twinkies as you would eating the same amount of lean protein, vegetables, fruit, and whole grains (for proof, see the "Cutting Calories Any Way You Please" box on page 9). Other health problems arise when you dedicate your diet to junk food, but we'll get into that later. The bottom line is that when it comes to weight loss—just weight loss—it's simple math. Eat fewer calories than you burn, and you will lose weight.

Marion Nestle, professor of human nutrition at New York University, inspired much of the Tiny and Full™ philosophy that I now believe to be the best method for losing weight. In her book, *Why Calories Count*, she uses studies to show that cutting calories is the only reliable method for reducing weight. This is not a new idea. The whole idea of what a calorie is—a measurement of the energy, heat, or work in a food, or the energy or work that is expended in physical activity—was discovered and solidified in the 1800s. Scientists have long understood that to maintain weight, you must have a balance between the number of calories you consume and the number you expend. To lose weight, you must consume less food than you expend, or you must expend more calories in exercise than you consume in food. What you eat doesn't really matter in this equation. Consider these studies:

- In a study published in the *Journal of the American Dietetic Association*, nutrition researchers from Texas Woman's University found that regardless of the components of a diet, as long as the participants stuck to the calorie restrictions, they lost weight. The study separated women into three groups of at least 11 per group and had them eat 1,200-calorie diets of 25, 45, or 75 percent of carbohydrates with variations on fats and protein.

- In a 2001 review, researchers from the US Department of Agriculture and the University of California compared the high-protein, low-carb Atkins diet; the low-fat, high-carb Ornish plan; and the low-fat, moderate-carbohydrate Weight Watcher program. The study found that all three resulted in equal weight loss as long as the calories didn't exceed 1,400 to 1,500 calories per day. The researchers concluded that the major determinant of weight loss was calorie balance. All people succeed at losing

# On My Revelation

I have not recommended fruit for years due to its sugar calories, but I've discovered new research that has opened my eyes to how we look at food in relation to weight loss. As I continue to do research, I can't help but find indisputable evidence that there is another approach to weight loss that is more effective than just focusing on sugar calories. And today I am happily enjoying bowls full of watermelon and am leaner than I've ever been before.

"Sugar calories" is the term I used in my books *The 100* and *Happy Hormones, Slim Belly,* to define any carbohydrate calorie. It's an accurate term in that all carbohydrates are "read" as sugar by your body—hence sugar calories. The mistake I made was to say that all sugar calories are equal. They aren't. There are good sugars and bad sugars. The second misstep I took was following the advice of writers such as Gary Taubes, who argued persuasively that it was carbohydrate calories that caused weight gain. The truth is that too many calories cause weight gain, whatever food components they come from.

Knowledge exists in a flowing and changing state, and this includes nutrition and weight-loss research. Remember, once upon a time, we thought the world was flat. Several explorers were brave enough to venture out farther and discover the truth. In a similar vein, I have never believed in resting on my laurels. When I discover that I can share a better message for weight loss and health, I am always willing to update my philosophy to reflect the latest and most accurate science available. So, after much research, thought, and even internal struggle over accepting this science, I now have no lingering doubts that the most effective approach to weight loss is to consider all calories. That's it. All calories count.

Do I still think it's important to avoid refined sugars and flours? Absolutely. It's a great first step and vital to your health. However, just avoiding these empty calories won't cause weight loss in the way I once believed it would. I have discovered that "counting only sugar calories," along with the research relating to insulin and its effects on fat accumulation, is not as critical a factor to weight loss as watching your overall calories. In fact, it's actually quite insignificant.

So, I bring this information to you with the sincere hope that you will continue to trust me to bring you the latest dietary science and the most effective ways to lose weight and improve your health.

Here's to a big bowl of watermelon, grapes, and strawberries! You'll soon learn all about celebrating the one natural source of sweetness that will help you get the Tiny Waist you've always dreamed of having—and you'll find that fruit is an essential part of feeling Full while being Tiny!

weight when they eat fewer calories than they burn, regardless of protein, fat, or carbohydrate levels. In addition, the subjects all reported similar effects on hunger and satisfaction despite the diet followed.

- In a 2009 study published in *The New England Journal of Medicine*, researchers compared four diets: low fat, average protein; low fat, high protein; high fat, average protein; and high fat, high protein. Nearly 80 percent of the 200 people followed the dietary restrictions, all of which required the men and women to cut 750 calories off their daily intake. At the end of six months, the participants, regardless of diet group, had lost an average of nine pounds. All groups reported equal levels of hunger and diet satisfaction, and all had similar improvements in insulin and cholesterol. Because the weight loss was low and the calorie cutting was high, the investigators revisited the results and concluded that most participants had only reduced their calories by 250 per day. (The participants self-recorded their calories.)

As you can see, it doesn't matter *how* you cut calories—as long as you do. For some even more extreme diet examples, see the "Cutting Calories Any Way You Please" box on page 9.

In the next chapter, I'll explain all about bringing health into Tiny and Full™, but for now, I'm focusing on just the aspect of losing weight—nothing else. It's an important concept to understand. One thing we have plenty of in our society is constant access to plenty of highly nutritious foods. What we lack is moderation, and in regards to weight loss, moderation is the central concern.

## THE Problem: Hunger!

The central problem when it comes to cutting calories—what you need to do to get Tiny—is hunger! Your body does not like to be denied food. If you are deprived of calories, you'll want food and you'll want it right *now*. You'll be so bombarded with hunger signals incessantly telling you to eat that you'll become increasingly irritated, aggressive, and even angry. This concept is so common and pervasive that the term "hangry," an amalgam of "hungry" and "angry," has been added to the *Oxford Dictionaries* to describe this phenomenon of being bad-tempered, agitated, or irritable as a result of being hungry. You might even get hangry regularly, or love someone who does. Interestingly, a natural brain chemical, the neuropeptide Y that is released when you are hungry, is the same chemical your brain secretes when you feel angry or aggressive. This reaction is thought to be part of your evolutionary being that developed to protect you from going without food for too long. We didn't always have the plentiful open access to food that we have today. Back in the days of the hunter-gatherer, humans had to be prepared for times when food was scarce. Being aggressive and greedy about food was key to survival, which is why we don't act with grace when we are hangry. So while it isn't always pretty, hanger makes sense. Think about it. If our caveman forefather had been chill about the freshly killed wildebeest he worked so hard to hunt and had graciously invited the folks from the neighboring cave clan to join himself and his family, he and his might have starved. Being greedy and ravenous isn't our most civilized behavior, but when you are in a state of hanger, it's understandable.

Your body is a magnificent machine that is always working to maintain balance. Hunger is simply a signal to your body that it's out of balance. The feeling is unpleasant for a good reason. What you feel when you are deprived of food is your brain beckoning your body to eat. When you diet by cutting calories from your daily allotment, you naturally feel hungrier. Let's say you have a smaller breakfast than usual and you plan on having your lunch at the midday hour just like you normally do—only this time you are functioning on less than your average amount of calories (and remember, you'll be eating a smaller lunch portion as well). Your body takes notice of such things. As time passes since your last meal, the nutrients in your bloodstream (your blood glucose) begin to drop. If the drop is far enough, your brain will see it as an emergency situation. Initially, you feel the pangs of hunger, and you might get a headache, snarl at someone, or grow weak and fatigued. You might begin to have trouble concentrating. Your thoughts will increasingly turn to food, and you'll begin to obsess about when you can eat. Eventually, you'll be able to think of nothing else. The result in almost every circumstance is that you will eat. Now, if you are really pumped up about losing some weight and cutting calories, you might be able to stick to your plan for a few days, but being hungry day in and day out gets old pretty fast.

One survey from the UK found that women start about three different diets per year and quit on or around day 19. Yep. According to the researchers, by day 5, two-thirds had already cheated on their weight-loss plan. In another poll conducted by British researchers, 1,000 women reported that they quit their diets by week 5. As early as week 2, 25 percent had quit, and 50 percent dropped out by week 4. Not one woman reached her goal.

The other problem that comes with cutting calories is that your body's calorie-burning engine (your metabolism) slows down in proportion to the calories you cut and also to the weight you lose. If you want to continue to lose weight, you have to eat fewer and fewer calories as the number on the scale goes down; otherwise, you won't continue to lose weight. As time goes on, this gets tiresome, and, eventually, most of us bag the diet and overeat. Or, we diet for a certain amount of time, thinking that when we reach our goal, we'll get to splurge and eat again. And when you splurge, the weight comes back with a vengeance. Remember, your body thinks you've been starving it, so it greedily replaces whatever you've lost—and fast. This situation is why yo-yo dieting is as common as rain in Seattle. Consider the following studies that illustrate the common struggles with calorie cutting and hunger:

- In a Minnesota study, researchers put 19 men on a severe calorie-restricted diet, largely composed of potatoes. At the end of the six-month study, the men had become lethargic, depressed, irritable, cold, and lost all libido while they were eating a diet that severely limited their calories. They were constantly obsessed with thoughts of food. Their muscles grew weak, their endurance declined dramatically, and they lost muscle mass.

- In a study that examined the heart health of 18 voluntary calorie-restricting, antiaging enthusiasts, researchers at Washington University in St. Louis found that while they were about 20 percent leaner and had lower blood pressure, cholesterol, and markers of inflammation than a comparison group of "normal" eaters, the calorie restrictors were open about other difficulties. These members of the Calorie Restriction Society, who believe that the choice to reduce calorie intake will extend their life spans, report constant experiences of hunger and feeling cold. Women report menstrual irregularities, testosterone levels will decrease in men, and many say that they obsess about food and alienate family members and friends with their lifestyle choices.

- Of dieters who lose weight, 80 to 95 percent gain it back within a year or two, according to a 2010 National Health and Nutrition Examination Survey. Researchers speculate that cutting calories too severely, or following a rigid diet that cuts out certain food groups entirely, make most diets unsustainable and leave dieters too hungry. It's better to focus on avoiding highly processed foods and to eat moderately.

- In a Columbia University study, researchers underfed men and women to make them lose 10 to 20 percent of their weight. Not surprisingly, hunger increased while metabolism plummeted. After the studies ended, the subjects quickly regained the weight.

I have worked with many A-list stars who have horror stories of rigid self-starving plans they've put themselves on to lose weight. The dieting is miserable, and the weight loss is always temporary. It reminds me of the movie *The Devil Wears Prada*. While the movie is fictional, it's based on a true-life story of the fashion industry and how it glorifies the ultra-twiggy ideal for women. One of the all-too-real exchanges is between the editorial assistants Emily (played by Emily Blunt) and Andy Sachs (played by Anne Hathaway):

Emily: Andrea, my God! You look so chic.

Andy: Oh, thanks. You look so thin.

Emily: Really? It's for Paris. I'm on this new diet. Well, I don't eat anything, and when I feel like I'm about to faint, I eat a cube of cheese. I'm just one stomach flu away from my goal weight.

And another between the fashion director Nigel (played by Stanley Tucci) and Andy:

Andy: So none of the girls here eat anything?

Nigel: Not since two became the new four and zero became the new two.

Andy: Well, I'm a six . . .

Nigel: Which is the new fourteen.

These examples are unfortunately all too real for many women who want to achieve the ideal thinness factor. But it doesn't have to be this way. You don't have to starve or deprive yourself to have a Tiny Waist. You can be Tiny and Full™—and feel great having it all!

So how can you lose weight by cutting calories without suffering from feelings of deprivation and hunger? How can you counter the basic biological desire to eat that occurs when you restrict calories to lose weight? This is the weight-loss paradox—to get and maintain a Tiny Waist requires eating tiny amounts of food, which leads to being hangry and then, often, to binging and regaining weight. Being hungry or hangry obviously isn't the answer.

The good news is that I have a solution that works! There is no reason to suffer. You can actually feel Full and have a Tiny Waist. Feeling Full is not being stuffed like a Thanksgiving turkey. It's important to understand the difference. People who have dieted for decades have often lost touch with the internal signals the body gives to alert them to levels of satiation. Feeling Full, not uncomfortably stuffed, is the feeling of being satisfied, content, and *not* hungry. When you are a healthy "Full," you aren't thinking about food. You know that you have nourished yourself appropriately and don't need to eat again for a few hours. You could eat more, but if you did, you would cross from being Full to being uncomfortably bloated and distended. Being Full is being energized, comfortable, relaxed, and happy. Are you Ready for Full? Then, turn the page.

# Ready for Full

17

Are you ready to banish hunger and deprivation forever? You may believe that the only way to lose weight, the only way to get a Tiny Waist, is to starve yourself and to suffer the pangs of hunger and deprivation—but that isn't true. If you have a long history of dieting, it might seem impossible, but you are about to learn that you can have both—a Tiny Waist and a Full belly. In the previous chapter, I explained the necessity of creating a calorie deficit (eating fewer calories than you burn) for weight loss, but that doesn't mean that you have to feel like you are starving. In fact, you can feel Full at all times. There is a better way, and that's what you'll learn in these next pages. Getting Ready for Full means absorbing the knowledge outlined in this chapter. After you've read these pages, you'll never have to feel starved or deprived again. You'll never again find yourself *off* a diet binging because you're ravenous, and you'll never again go *on* a depriving diet struggling for a slim waist because Tiny and Full™ isn't a diet that you go *on* or *off*. It's a lifestyle plan that you'll love so much, you'll never have to think about dieting again.

## What is Full?

Being Full is both a way of eating and a frame of mind. When it comes to eating, the concept of Full is about being satisfied, not stuffed. This will be our main focus. I'm going to teach you how to take practical steps to eat so you are always satisfied. Never again will you feel ravenous or restricted.

The other perspective of Full, just like with Tiny in the previous chapter, is having a mind-set of Full. Being "Full of mind" means being filled with vitality, energy, wisdom, knowledge, confidence, happiness, and peace. When someone says, "I have a full life," isn't that what they mean? Having a Full mind-set can also be applied to your attitude in regards to food and eating. Knowing that you deserve to eat healthy foods that nourish you and propel you to become Tiny is having a Full attitude about your style of eating. Being Full, in this sense, means that you don't have to worry about eating or have to think of food as something to fear, restrict, or forbid. When I say you are going to eat Full, I am saying that you are going to eat a balanced diet packed with nutrients, vitamins, minerals, and antioxidants, but this is not a food plan that is devoid of empty or harmful calories (I'll explain more in the next section).

To bring this concept together, I want you to understand that having a Full life means being *Full*-filled in all areas of your life, as well as being free and confident to accomplish everything on your life's bucket list. Plus, Full goes hand in hand with Tiny. If you remember from the previous chapter, when you are Tiny, you are beautiful inside and out—because being beautiful on the outside is an exterior reflection of your interior health. Being Full, in your attitude and in your style of eating, is how you will get to be Tiny. When your life is *Full*, you will be Tiny—and when you are *Tiny*, your life will be Full. Put both together, and you will be filled with epic health, serenity, happiness, and confidence.

Now, let's move on to the nutritional aspect of how to eat to always feel Full, but not overstuffed or starving.

Ready?

Three things:

1. Calorie density: To get you FULL-ly prepared to be Full, first we need to discuss the concept of calorie density so you'll understand how to choose foods to be Tiny, while never feeling hungry or deprived again.

2. Optimal eating: We'll explore how veganism maximizes low calorie density and boosts your health so you can always be Full. These strategies for Full Eating to get a Tiny Waist will help you to never feel deprived or hungry.

3. The problem: Eating vegan all day, every day, deprives you of vital nutrients and is not sustainable. We'll explore the shortcomings of veganism.

By the end of this chapter, you'll have both components of what it takes to be Tiny and Full™. You will effortlessly create a new lifestyle you can follow with ease! You will be free, once and for all, from yo-yo dieting, gimmicks, and fad diets, and you'll have the clarity and focus you need to reach the freedom, health, and beauty you've always desired.

# Not All Foods Will Fill You Equally

In the previous chapter, Ready for Tiny, I shared how I've come to a new understanding, based on overwhelming research, that to be truly and forever Tiny, you must watch your overall calorie intake. This presents a problem—hunger. Your body is incredibly sensitive to the calories it is accustomed to getting on a daily basis. When you cut calories, it makes you feel hungry, which can set up a dangerous reaction of overeating. You might be able to stick to a reduced-calorie plan for a few weeks, but when you feel empty from the lack of calories you are used to having, it becomes increasingly difficult to stick to your goal to get that Tiny Waist. Obsessive thoughts about food, irritability, and hunger eventually win.

Fortunately, there is a simple and clear solution—being Full! I'm not being flippant here, because there is a trustworthy method that you can use to plan your meals and to eat foods that will keep you satisfied, while cutting calories so you can get Tiny. The secret to being steadily Full while lowering your calorie intake begins with understanding that not all foods are created equal. While a calorie is always a calorie, some foods are more *calorie dense* than others. What does that mean? A calorie-dense food has lots of calories, or energy, packed into a relatively small package. Let's take a closer look at this essential concept.

## What is calorie density?

Barbara Rolls, nutrition professor and researcher at Penn State and author of *The Ultimate Volumetrics Diet,* coined the term "calorie density" to describe how foods vary in the number of calories they pack into each bite. Calorie density refers to the number of calories (or the amount of energy) contained in a gram of food. Foods with a lower calorie density provide fewer calories per gram than foods with a higher calorie density. Basically, for the same amount of calories, you can eat a larger portion of a food that is low in calorie density than of a food that is high in calorie density. For example, let's say you'd like to eat a snack of about 150 calories. If you choose a small bag of Doritos from your office vending machine (a high-calorie-density food), you can have 11 chips to reach this quota. However, if you decide to have a bowl of strawberries (a low-calorie-density food), you can have 37 strawberries for the same 150 calories. Not only do the portion sizes look dramatically different—barely a handful of chips versus an overflowing bowl of juicy fruit—the first snack offers you nothing but salt, sugar, and empty calories that won't fill you up at all, while strawberries are low in fat and full of all-natural flavors and colors, fiber, minerals, antioxidants, and vitamins (for more examples of calorie density and how it affects portion size, see the following picture of the varying sizes of 100-calorie snacks).

# Which would you choose?

Here's what 100 calories of different snacks looks like. You can eat any of these and still eat the same amount of calories, but which ones do you think would fill you up the most?

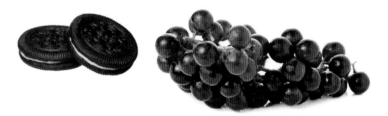

2 Oreo cookies (100 calories) or 62 grapes (100 calories)

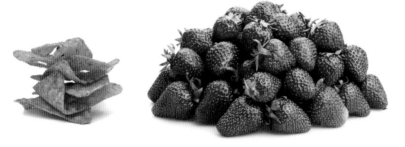

8 Dorito chips (100 calories) or 25 medium strawberries (100 calories)

Eating these lower-calorie-density foods isn't a trick—you are actually filling your stomach with more food (by volume or weight), but you eat far fewer calories. That is calorie density in action. And it works! Researchers from the University of Alabama at Birmingham, Harvard, Spain, and many others, along with the Penn State researchers led by Rolls, have conducted a wealth of studies that show that lowering the calorie density of foods helps you to feel Full while eating fewer calories. Again and again, this research shows that you can lose weight while keeping your belly consistently and steadily Full. Consider these examples:

- Stay Full, eat less, be Tiny: Researchers from the Centers for Disease Control and Prevention conducted a survey of more than 7,000 adults and found that when compared to those who ate high-calorie-density foods, those who ate larger amounts of low-calorie-density foods ate fewer calories overall, even though they ate more food by weight. Remember, low-calorie-density foods fill up your plate, and your belly, without filling you with the calories that cause weight gain. This study, published in *The American Journal of Clinical Nutrition,* found that people with diets highest in fruits and vegetables (the lowest-calorie-density foods) ate the least calories and had the lowest rates of obesity.

- Size matters: In a study published in *Physiology & Behavior,* researchers from Pennsylvania State University and the Bell Institute of Health and Nutrition found that volume matters more than calorie count. For three days, the researchers had 36 women consume varying formulas of a milk-based liquid food—496 calories in 10 ounces (a little over a cup), 987 calories in 20 ounces (nearly three cups), or 496 calories in 20 ounces (also nearly three cups). The three milk drinks varied based on volume (size; some were larger than others) and calorie density (the amount of calories per gram of drink; some had more calories than others). All drinks tasted similar and had the same nutrient composition. The women all rated the drinks as tasting similar and being equally enjoyable, but how satisfying—*how Full*—each drink made the woman feel was directly related to how large the drink was. The largest drink for the least calories was just as satisfying as the largest drink with the most calories. Again—you can be Full on less.

- Cut calories effortlessly: In another study, jointly published by Pennsylvania State University, the University of Alabama at Birmingham, Pennington Biomedical Research Center, Kaiser Permanente, Duke University, and Johns Hopkins Medical Center, researchers found that successful weight loss occurred when calorie density was reduced. When more than 650 overweight and obese men and women were divided into three groups, those who ate the lowest-calorie-density foods consumed the least calories, compared to groups that had higher-calorie-density foods. It gets even more impressive when you consider that compared to the highest-calorie-density diet group, the lowest-calorie-density diet group lost the most weight (5.3 pounds in the high-density group versus 13 pounds in the low-density group). The low-calorie-density group also decreased their calorie intake per day more (500 for the low-calorie-density group, while the high-calorie-density group only cut 100 calories per day). Plus, the low-calorie-density group increased the weight of the food they ate per day by 300 grams, while the high-calorie-density group didn't change the weight significantly at all. Again, this means that the people eating the low-calorie-density foods visually saw more food on their plates and felt more food in their bellies, while eating an average of 500 calories less a day than the high-calorie-density group did.

- Let them eat soup!: In a trial with 200 overweight men and women, researchers at Penn State, led by Rolls, tested the effect of incorporating either a low-calorie-density food or a high-calorie-density food into a reduced-calorie diet. The study found that reducing calorie density by adding a low-calorie-density soup into the diets of men and women was the main predictor of weight loss during the first two months of the study. Did you get that? The researchers *added* a food—the low-calorie-density soup, which was basically vegetables in broth—and that alone helped the subjects who had soup to lose weight. In addition, this strategy increased the amount of weight lost and the success at maintaining the loss.

- Eat more veggies and fruits: In another Penn State study, Rolls and colleagues tested the effect of lowering calorie density on a group of 97 obese women. The first group was directed to increase the amount of water-rich foods, such as vegetables and fruits, and to lower fat. The second group was told to restrict portions and to reduce fat. A year later, the group told to eat more fruits and vegetables had a greater reduction in calorie density and lost more weight than the group told to simply restrict portions. I love this positive strategy. Instead of telling the participants to cut foods, the researchers told them to eat *more* fruits and vegetables—and the group that was told to eat more lost the weight!

Our goal is to mimic the research you've just read about to eat the most nutrient-rich, but calorie-light foods to maintain a constant feeling of fullness while creating a calorie deficit that results in steady and sustainable weight and fat loss.

How will we do this?

Let's get to it.

## Bulking up the portions

What makes the biggest difference in portion sizes are water and air. The quality of being filling also comes from fiber in foods, but that won't necessarily change the portion size. The examples given so far have been foods that have more water (and vitamins, fiber, minerals, and antioxidants), but you can also achieve this same effect, of larger portions, by whipping in, or whipping up, various meals, which you'll learn about in later chapters (think yummy smoothies and shakes). Weight-loss researchers say this is an important concept because what you see affects how Full you feel. The previous research examples all provide proof that this is true. The research by Rolls and her colleagues emphasizes that we all hold inherent beliefs about how much food we need to see on our plates or in our bowls to feel satisfied. When you see a full plate of food, your brain registers that you will be receiving enough nourishment, and you feel more satisfied. Once again, this shows that it's what you *see* on your plate that matters, not how many calories are *in* the food on your plate. This is good news because it means you can eat a low-calorie, highly nutritious meal and be sufficiently Full. The result is weight loss without ever feeling hungry or deprived.

## Understanding the calorie density of various foods

All foods are made up of a blend of various macronutrients—fat, carbohydrates, protein, water, fiber, and sometimes alcohol. Combined, these components determine the calories in a given food and the calorie density (see the image on the following page). It's helpful to look at each macronutrient separately to see where calorie density of a food is highest:

- Fat has 9 calories per gram, making it the most calorie dense of all macronutrients.

- Alcohol has 7 calories per gram and rates almost as high as fat. Alcohol is a special commodity as well because it isn't metabolized like other foods. Based on this, it should be consumed sparingly.

- Both protein and carbohydrates (including all sugars) come in at 4 calories per gram.

- Fiber, while also a carbohydrate, is only partially digestible, and so it comes in at 2 calories per gram.

- Water is the one and only true "free" nutrient because it has 0 calories, and 0 calorie density. It adds weight and volume without any calories—so the "wetter" the better. The more water in a food means the more food you'll see on your plate, in your bowl, or filling your cup.

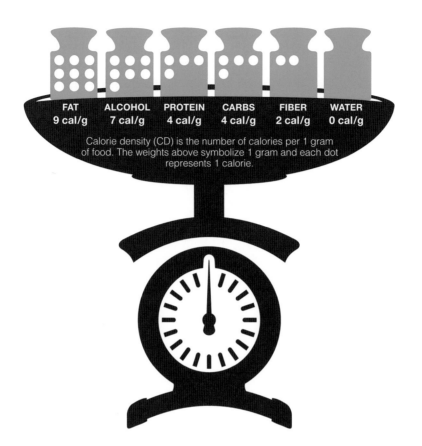

Calorie density (CD) is the number of calories per 1 gram of food. The weights above symbolize 1 gram and each dot represents 1 calorie.

| FAT | ALCOHOL | PROTEIN | CARBS | FIBER | WATER |
|-----|---------|---------|-------|-------|-------|
| 9 cal/g | 7 cal/g | 4 cal/g | 4 cal/g | 2 cal/g | 0 cal/g |

## How to calculate calorie density

You can calculate the calorie density of any food. Simply turn to the nutrition label of any package of food in your kitchen (or look it up nonpackaged items on calorieking.com), and look for the serving size and the calories per serving. Let's consider a 5-ounce single serving of plain, nonfat Greek yogurt. The serving size in grams is 130, and the calorie per serving is 90. To calculate the calorie density, divide the calories per serving by the grams per serving. Here, 90 divided by 130 is .69, meaning that the calorie density of this yogurt is .69.

Calories per serving ÷ Grams per serving = Calorie density per serving

or

90 ÷ 130 = .69

You can get a reasonable idea of how calorie dense a food is by using this calculation on any food and then using the following chart as a guide.

# Hunger Signals:
# When to Start Eating and When to Stop

One key part of being Tiny and Full™ is to understand your hunger and fullness signals. If you've been following one diet plan or another over the past several years, you've likely lost the ability to listen to the small quiet voice inside that tells you when to start eating and when to stop eating. When you are starving, that inner voice isn't so quiet—it screams. Ditto for when you are stuffed. The problem is that if you wait until your body is shrieking for food or wailing because you are bloated beyond comfort, it's too late. The damage is done, and you're either going to be inhaling food like a thousand-dollar Dyson, or you're going to be in agony, popping Tums all night and beating yourself up for going overboard. That's why you have to learn to listen for the subtler signals. Start making use of the following scale right away to help you get back in touch with your hunger and full signals.

Throughout the day, check in and see how you are feeling on a hunger or fullness level. Rate your hunger on the scale of 1 to 10. You want to aim to eat when you are at a 3–4 and to stop when you are around 5–6.

1—Ravenous, weak, dizzy, jittery, headache; hangry. Can't concentrate. Stomach acid is churning. You don't care what you eat, but you must eat—now!

2—Stomach growling, cranky, feel a headache coming on, can't stop thinking about food.

3—Stomach is starting to growl, stomach feels empty, eating would be enjoyable now.

4—Could eat something, may feel the first pangs or gurgles of hunger; you notice your first thoughts of food.

5—Full, satisfied, neither hungry nor full; your stomach doesn't feel bloated at all.

6—Perfectly and pleasantly full, relaxed, and comfortable.

7—Starting to feel a little uncomfortable. Food stops tasting as good. Stomach feels a bit stretched. You start to feel sleepy.

8—Need to unbutton your pants; you know you've gone too far, and you feel regret.

9—Your stomach hurts, feeling heavy and uncomfortable; clothes feel tight.

10—You are so overstuffed it hurts. You are in a food coma. You feel sick. You are Thanksgiving-dinner full.

# The Tiny and Full™ Levels

## Level 1

How to Eat: Fill up on these foods as much as possible. These should be your "go-to" food choices.

Examples: Non-starchy vegetables, most fruits, and broth-based soups

## Level 2

How to Eat: Eat reasonable portions from this level.

Examples: Lean protein, legumes, low-fat dairy

## Level 3

How to Eat: Add Level 3 when necessary, but make sure to manage your portions.

Examples: Breads, desserts, cheeses, higher-fat meats

## Level 4

How to Eat: Limit Level 4 as much as possible, and make sure to watch your portions and frequency of eating.

Examples: Fried snacks, candy, cookies, nuts, fat, wine

Quick Tip: If the number of grams per serving of a food is larger than the calories per serving, the food is a low-calorie-density food, and you can safely include it in your diet.

However, you won't have to worry about calculating the calorie density of the foods you'll be eating. I've done all the work for you in the Tiny and Full™ Foods list in Chapter 7 as well as this quick-reference guide (see next page) of foods that fall in the four Tiny and Full™ levels:

# The Tiny and Full™ Levels

## Level 1

**Plant-Based Food**

Soups

Tomato soup, prepared with water
Black bean soup, prepared with water
Lentil soup

Vegetables

Cucumber
Spinach, raw
Zucchini, steamed
Broccoli, raw
Green beans, cooked
Bell pepper, red, raw

Fruits

Watermelon
Strawberries
Grapefruit
Blackberries
Orange
Pineapple, raw
Raspberries
Blueberries

**Animal-Based Food**

Soups

Chicken noodle soup
Vegetable beef soup
Lentil and ham soup
Chicken tortilla soup

Dairy

Milk, fat-free
Yogurt, Greek, nonfat, plain
Yogurt, nonfat, plain

Mixed Dishes

Shake, pea, prepared with water

## Level 2

**Plant-Based Food**

Soups

Chunky vegetable
Split pea

Vegetables, Legumes (Beans, Peas)

Sweet potato, baked or mashed
Green peas, cooked
Beans, kidney
Beans, Lima, cooked
Corn, boiled, drained

Fruits

Mango
Grapes
Banana

Cereals, Grains

Rice, wild, cooked
Rice, brown, long-grain, cooked
Quinoa, cooked

**Animal-Based Food**

Soups

Clam chowder, prepared with milk
Chunky bean with ham soup

Dairy

Milk, Whole
Yogurt, low-fat, plain
Yogurt, low-fat, fruit
Cream cheese, fat-free

Meat, Poultry, Fish

Tuna, light, canned in water
Tilapia, cooked
Turkey breast, roasted, no skin
Ham, extra lean

Condiments

Sour cream, regular
Ranch dressing, fat-free

## Level 3

**Plant-Based Food**

Vegetables, Legumes (Beans, Peas)
  Hummus
  Potatoes, French-fried

Fruits
  Avocado, California
  Raisins

Breads
  Tortilla, corn
  Pita, whole-wheat
  Bread, white
  Bread, whole-grain

Desserts, Snack Foods
  Hard pretzels

**Animal-Based Food**

Dairy
  Cream cheese, light
  Cheese, feta
  Mozzarella cheese, part skim
  Cheese, Swiss, reduced fat

Meat, Poultry, Fish, Eggs
  Chicken breast, roasted, no skin
  Egg, hard-boiled
  Sirloin steak, lean, broiled
  Salmon, farmed, baked
  Pork chop, center loin, broiled
  Ground beef, lean, broiled

Mixed Dishes
  Cheese pizza, thin crust
  Cheeseburger, fast food
  Biscuit with egg and sausage

Desserts, Snack Foods
  Frozen yogurt, soft serve
  Ice cream, premium

Condiments
  Mayonnaise, light

## Level 4

**Plant-Based Food**

Breads, Crackers
  Wheat crackers

Desserts, Snack Foods, Candy
  Popcorn, caramel
  Brownie
  Donut, cake
  Trail mix
  Potato chips, baked
  Potato chips, regular
  Tortilla chips, regular
  Granola bar, hard
  Chocolate, dark

Nuts
  Peanut butter, reduced-fat
  Almonds, dry-roasted
  Peanuts, roasted
  Peanut butter, regular
  Pecans, dry-roasted

Condiments
  Berry jam
  Oil, olive

**Animal-Based Food**

Dairy
  Cheese, Parmesan
  Butter

Meat
  Pork spareribs, braised
  Bacon, cooked

Desserts, Snack Foods, Candy
  Carrot cake, cream cheese frosting
  Brownie
  Chocolate chip cookies, homemade

Condiments
  Oil, olive

# Optimizing Low-Calorie-Density Eating

So now you know all about the science of calorie density, and it makes sense. Still, it can be challenging to stick to this strategy all day every day. Of course, I've found the perfect solution—don't I always? What's the best way to low-calorie-density eating and staying Full, losing weight, and getting that Tiny Waist? My investigation of the facts led me again and again to see that the most purely vegetarian diet, a vegan diet, is the way to go.

You will also want to know how to prepare foods to give you the fullest portions and nutrients while having the lowest calories. The simplest way to achieve this is to use high-calorie-density foods as condiments and low-calorie-density foods as the foundation of all meals and snacks. Envision breakfasts of brightly colored fruit salads—strawberries, watermelon, blueberries, mangoes, melons—topped with a smattering of sliced almonds, sunflower seeds, or pepitas. Or you might have a large frothy fruit shake made with pea protein, whipped up with ice to fill a

## Are you getting enough water?

They used to say "drink eight 8oz. glasses of water a day." However, to think that such a blanket statement should work for all different shapes and sizes seems a little off.

How much water you need really depends on your height, weight, as well as how active you are and even where you live! A good rule of thumb is that you need between 0.5-1oz. of water for every 1 lb. you weigh...every day. For example, if you weigh 140 lbs., you should be drinking between 70-140oz of water daily. If you workout a lot or live in a hotter area, you will need to be closer to the 140oz range. If you are more sedentary and live in cooler climates, you are safe to be somewhere in the middle or towards the lower end.

Use these tips to get more water in each day.

- Use the Tiny and Full bottle - holds 20oz - and fill it up throughout the day.

- Drink more than one cup of coffee? Swap one cup for a glass of water.

- Spread your water consumption out throughout the day. Drinking a lot of water all at once is not good for you.

- Keep glasses or bottles of water on your desk, by your bed, and anywhere else where you will be reminded to take a sip!

large glass. Lunches can be stir-fried zucchini, carrots, snow peas, and celery with small portions of lean chicken or fish on top. A large chef or spinach salad or a veggie-based casserole is on tap for dinner. These are all simple ways to add bulk without the calories.

## It's all about veganism

Did you notice that many of these strategies are also vegan? That's because eating a vegan diet is the one best option for superior health and for eating a low-calorie-density diet. It isn't as daunting as it sounds, and vegans are fundamentally healthier. Let's take a closer look at what it means to eat vegan.

## The benefits of eating vegan

More and more people are turning to a vegan diet for the health benefits. Vegans report increased energy, better mood and mind-set, weight loss, and younger-looking skin. The scientific research on people who eat the most fruits and vegetables and

# What about alcohol?

100 proof alcohol has 7 calories per gram. That's pretty high, especially since it won't fill you up. It's important to think of alcohol, and any beverages with calories, and "empty calories." Calories that count, but don't help you feel full.

So, while it is not recommended that you drink your calories, I understand that sometimes we like to enjoy a cocktail or glass of wine. I'm right there with you! Here are my tips for doing it without messing up your day.

1—Remember that calories count, so make sure to stay within your daily caloric goal.

2—Replace your 100 calorie treat at the end of the night with 100 calories of the following:

- 1 glass red wine
- 9 oz. vodka soda
- 12.5 oz light beer
- 4 oz. red or white wine (note, this is less than a typical pour of wine)
- 5 oz. Bloody Mary
- 1.5 oz or 1 shot of liquor

# The Natural Nutrient Benefits of Eating Vegan

In addition to being naturally lower in calorie density, the following nutrients are inherently more present in vegan diets:

- **Fiber:** Dietary fiber includes all parts of plant foods that your body can't digest or absorb. Fiber passes pretty much intact through your digestive tract. Why is this good? Fiber helps your body lower blood cholesterol and blood sugar levels, helps you have regular and painless bowel movements, and has been shown to lower the risk of cancers, heart disease, type 2 diabetes, and obesity. Fiber-rich foods include navy beans, pinto beans, kidney beans, lentils, black beans, prunes, pears, mangoes, almonds, pistachios, and pumpkin.

- **Folic acid:** Folic acid is a B vitamin that helps your body make healthy new cells. Both men and women need folic acid, but it's particularly important to women before and during pregnancy because it helps prevent major birth defects. Folic acid keeps your blood healthy and protects you from anemia; it's also been shown to increase heart health and protect against cell changes that can cause cancer. Foods rich in folic acid include lentils, beans, peas, dark green vegetables, okra, asparagus, and citrus fruits.

- **Vitamin C:** This is one of the most powerful and effective nutrients, and with all the vegetables and fruits vegans eat, they get plenty of it. Vitamin C is necessary for the growth, development, and repair of all body tissues. Scientific studies of vitamin C show that it reduces stress, reduces the duration and intensity of the common cold, protects against stroke risk, guards eyesight, reduces overall inflammation, decreases cancer risk, protects your heart, and even slows the aging process of your skin. Vitamin C boosts the body's ability to absorb iron, enhances the immune system, increases wound healing, and helps in the maintenance of bones, teeth, and cartilage. This vitamin is also considered an antioxidant for its role as protector against free radicals and toxins such as cigarette smoke. Most fruits offer an excellent source of vitamin C, as do some vegetables, including tomatoes; red, yellow, and orange bell peppers; dark leafy greens; broccoli; and more.

- **Vitamin E:** In the past few years, the information about the benefits of taking vitamin E as a supplement has become unclear. However, vitamin E in foods such as almonds, hazelnuts, seeds, Swiss chard, spinach, and kale is safe and shown to be key for strong immunity, strong vision, and healthy skin.

- **Potassium:** This mineral is part of every cell in your body, and it helps your cells to function properly. It helps your nerves and muscles to communicate, assists in the regulation and maintenance of healthy blood pressure, and plays a vital role in helping your heart to beat properly. Healthy vegans eat plenty of potassium-rich foods such as dark leafy greens, potatoes, squash, avocados, mushrooms, and bananas. If you find yourself overly tired, irritable, or grumpy, it could be a sign that your potassium is too low. Other signs of low potassium include cramping, feelings of overall weakness, and nausea.

- **Magnesium:** I've written about magnesium before. It's an essential nutrient for many reasons, but one reason that caught my attention recently was in a study in *The Journal of Intensive Care Medicine,* which reported that being deficient in magnesium doubles your risk of dying compared to those who have sufficient magnesium. Besides this attention-grabbing research, magnesium has long been known to reduce stress and enhance relaxation. Magnesium also reduces the risk of insomnia, eases cramps, boosts mood, keeps kidneys healthy, and has been associated with reducing chronic diseases such as heart disease, diabetes, osteoporosis, and certain cancers. Magnesium-rich foods include almonds, dark leafy greens, peas, nuts, and whole grains.

- **Phytochemicals:** These biologically active compounds in plants are made up of several beneficial properties, including antioxidants. Scientists are still learning the benefits of these naturally occurring compounds, but they believe them to be largely responsible for the protective health benefits in plant-based foods. Phytonutrients are found in fruits, vegetables, whole grains, legumes, herbs, spices, nuts, and seeds.

## What It Really Means to Be Vegan

When I say "vegan," I mean in the truest, most natural form of vegan. A whole food (minimally processed), plant-based diet. A vegan can technically live on Coke, potato chips, and processed tofu dogs, but that is not the "vegan" I support. I encourage the healthiest, most natural form of vegan possible, which means eating whole, plant-based foods.

the least animal protein show that those on vegan-style diets have the lowest levels of chronic disease and longer life spans. The plant sources of these diets tend to be packed with nutrients but not calories. These diets are naturally higher in fiber, folic acid, vitamins C and E, potassium, magnesium, and phytochemicals, and they are lower in saturated fats (see "The Natural Nutrient Benefits of Eating Vegan" box on page 32). It's easy to see that eating vegan is a great strategy for eating low-calorie-density foods because, as I've already mentioned, the lowest-calorie-dense foods are plant foods—fruits and vegetables—and if you are vegan, that's all you'll be eating. These are also the foods that are the most jam-packed with nutrients, vitamins, minerals, fiber, and antioxidants. Not convinced? Check out just a sampling of the research on the benefits of going vegan:

- Boosts immunity and prevents disease: In a study published in the *Journal of the National Cancer Institute,* researchers from the Harvard School of Public Health found that of more than 100,000 men and women, those who ate the most fruits and vegetables (the most vegan diets) had lower rates of heart disease, cancer, and death of any type than those who ate the least fruits and vegetables.

- Protects your heart: A UK review study of dietary habits that analyzed 12 studies, including more than 278,000 men and women for 11 years, found that those who ate the highest levels of fruits and vegetables had the lowest rates of heart disease. The researchers, from St. George's University of London, determined that individuals who had fewer than three servings per day of fruit and vegetables had a 17 percent greater risk of heart disease or heart attacks than those who ate five or more servings of plant foods per day.

- Lowers stroke risk: In another review study by the same UK research group as above, investigators analyzed stroke risk among people and correlated it with fruit and vegetable consumption. Of the eight studies and more than 250,000 men and women that spanned the course of 13 years, the researchers found that individuals who ate fewer than three servings of fruit and vegetables per day had the highest risk of stroke compared to those who ate five or more servings of fruits and veggies per day. The protective effects of fruits and vegetables were so strong that they led the researchers to strongly advise eating a minimum of five servings per day.

- Keeps blood pressure low: In a *Journal of American Medical Association* review of 32 scientific studies, researchers from Japan, Pennsylvania, and Washington, DC, found that eating a vegetarian diet influenced healthy blood pressure. The researchers analyzed more than 21,000 men and women and found that those who ate a vegetarian diet reduced their average systolic blood pressure by nearly 7 mm/Hg and their average diastolic blood pressure by nearly 5 mm/Hg. Those who ate animal protein didn't lower their blood pressure. Another study that analyzed the effects of plant foods on blood pressure, published in *The New England Journal of Medicine*, found that when 459 men and women ate either a diet low in fruits and vegetables or a diet rich in fruits and vegetables for three weeks, those in the high plant food group lowered their blood pressure by 11.4 and 5.5 mm/Hg points. The low vegetable and fruit group didn't lower their blood pressure at all.

- Reduces bad cholesterol: In a Brazilian study, researchers from the Catholic University at São Paulo found that vegans had LDL cholesterol that was 44 percent lower than those who ate a traditional diet. The researchers collected blood samples from 76 men and women who were separated into groups according to diet styles (omnivores, lacto-ovo vegetarians, lacto vegetarians, and vegans).

- Reduces diabetes risk: In a study published in *Diabetes Care,* researchers followed more than 71,000 women, ages 38 to 63, for 18 years. During the follow-up phase of the study, the Tulane University researchers found that those who reported a diet high in fruit and leafy green vegetables had a lower rate of diabetes than those who didn't eat many plant foods. In addition, those women who reported high fruit juice consumption had an increased risk of diabetes. Fruit juice is really just an isolated and concentrated form of the fruit, but without the nutritional benefits.

- Protects your eyes: From a study of more than 39,000 women, Harvard researchers found that munching on fruits and vegetables preserves eye function. After the initial assessment, the researchers did a follow-up 10 years later and found that the women who had the highest intake of fruits and vegetables had a 10 to 15 percent lower risk of having cataracts than those who ate the lowest amounts of plant foods.

- Lowers cancer risk: Eating deep yellow and dark green fruits and vegetables and eating onions and garlic are all associated with a lower risk of colorectal cancer, according to a University at Buffalo, School of Public Health study reported in the *American Journal of Clinical Nutrition.* Using findings of more than 3,000 men and women who were screened for colorectal cancers and comparing them to more than 29,000 control subjects, the researchers detected a reduced risk for these types of cancers among those who had the lowest risk of cancers. In addition to this research, many experts who study vegan diets and cancer risks say that the high consumption of whole fruits, vegetables, and legumes provides a powerful and regular dosing of phytochemicals that protect against many cancers. As mentioned earlier, phytochemicals are the active compounds found in plant-based foods. Because vegans consume considerably more of the foods that have been shown in scientific research to be protective against many types of cancers—including legumes, total fruit and vegetables, tomatoes, allium vegetables, fiber, and vitamin C—it's reasonable to conclude that vegans are more highly protected from many types of cancers.

- Reduces the risk of weight gain: People who follow diets that are rich in vegetables and fruits are less likely to gain weight over the same time period than those who have diets scarce in plant foods. In a study published in the *American Journal of Clinical Nutrition,* researchers analyzed the data of more than 89,000 men and women from five countries. Those who ate the most fruits and vegetables had the lowest changes in weight. In another study from the journal *Nutrition* that followed the dietary patterns of more than 10,000 men and women for 10 years, researchers from the Department of Preventive Medicine and Public Health at the University of Navarra, Spain, found that those who consumed the most fruits and vegetables had the least weight gain, compared to those who didn't consume as many fruits and vegetables.

To sum it up: to eat vegan is to be healthy, slim, energized, happy, and confident. Unfortunately, there's a snag or two when it comes to being a full-time vegan.

# The Vegan Flaw

While the vegan diet is good for you and good for the world, there's a problem—or three. Vegans do have superior health benefits because of diets with higher amounts of fiber, folic acid, vitamins C and E, potassium, magnesium, many phytochemicals, and lower intake of saturated fats, but this style of eating also comes with potential health risks. Eating this way all day every day means missing out on key nutrients if you're not careful and being exposed to some health risks associated with veganism. Dealing with the rigidity and limiting quality of a full-time vegan lifestyle makes it unsustainable for the majority of people who attempt to follow the regimen. Celebrities from former president Bill Clinton to Beyoncé have tried the lifestyle and found it lacking.

Clinton explained to my good friend and celebrity chef Rachael Ray that he had to come to terms with the fact that he wasn't getting the quality protein and nutrients while eating a vegan diet. Clinton's doctor, Mark Hyman, expressed concern to the president, telling him, "It's hard being a vegan to eat enough good, quality protein, and not have too much starch. I know a lot of fat vegans." On the other side of celebrity-hood, diva-musician Beyoncé and her husband Jay Z recently launched a line of vegan meal plans. Beyoncé has said that she feels more energy and sees an enhanced glow to her skin from eating the vegan way, but admitted that she doesn't follow the strategy full time.

## Missing nutrients

Several key nutrients are often lacking in a vegan diet, including vitamins, minerals, and essential fatty acids. The nutritional adequacy of plant-based diets for weight management was recently discussed in great detail in a paper published in *The American Journal of Clinical Nutrition*. The review discusses information from the National Health and Nutrition Examination Survey (NHANES), a program of studies designed to assess the health and nutritional status of adults and children throughout the United States. The author concludes that while vegetarians and vegans do maintain healthier weights, they are at greater risk for deficiencies in vitamin B12, zinc, and protein as compared to those who eat animal protein. It's important to take a closer look at these nutrient risks and the health issues associated with them.

### Vitamin B12

Men and women need 2.4 mcg of this vitamin daily. Vitamin B12 is essential for having healthy blood cells and maintaining a healthy nervous system. A deficiency in this vitamin can cause abnormal neurologic and psychiatric symptoms that can include psychosis, nerve damage, disorientation, dementia, mood and motor disturbances, lack of energy, and difficulty concentrating. In a University of Wisconsin study, researchers tested the blood of 83 men and women who were attending the American Vegetarian Society Conference to determine vitamin B12 levels. The results of the study, published in the *Annals of Nutrition and Metabolism,* found that 92 percent of vegans were deficient in the vitamin, compared to lacto-vegetarians (47 percent were deficient) and semi-vegetarians (just 20 percent were deficient). B12 is found only in animal proteins, including eggs, poultry, beef, fish, and dairy products. Although some plant foods, including mushrooms, tempeh, miso, and sea vegetables, are reported to have some vitamin B12, they are not reliable. These foods contain an inactive form of the vitamin, and not only can it not be absorbed, it interferes with the absorption of active B12. Many vegans need to take a B12 supplement to maintain proper levels.

### Vitamin D

Vitamin D is known to be highly beneficial in protecting bone health and reducing the risk of heart disease, type 2 diabetes, high blood pressure, and cancer. The scientific evidence suggests that vegan populations often have low vitamin D levels, which is associated with an increased risk of some cancers. In an Oxford University study, researchers found that of more than 65,000 men and women, those who were vegans had the lowest levels of vitamin D, compared to all other eating styles. Compared to the meat eaters, the vegans' average vitamin D level was 75 percent lower. In another study, Finnish investigators followed the vitamin D status and bone health of 28 women for one year. The women were separated into three groups: vegans, lacto-vegetarians, and omnivores. Blood and urine samples were collected over the course of 12 months, and the vegans were found to have consistently lower levels of vitamin D and lower bone density than either the vegetarians or omnivores. The bone density in the vegans was 12 percent lower than in the omnivores.

### Iron

The daily iron quota for adult women, ages 18 to 50, is 18 mg. For men and for women after menopause (mid-50s for most), the daily requirement is 8 mg per day. Surprisingly, vegans do not show an increased risk for iron deficiency anemia, but they do tend to have lower iron stores. While you can get sufficient iron from dark leafy greens and beans in a vegan diet, it takes focus and work. Low iron increases your risk for anemia, a condition that can cause constant fatigue.

### Zinc

Meat, seafood, and animal products are high in zinc. Interestingly, many vegan foods tend to lower the absorption of zinc. Zinc is essential for metabolism, the immune system, and healing.

### Calcium

Adults ages 18 to 50 need 1,000 mg of calcium daily. Those over age 51 need 1,200 mg daily. Most of you know that calcium is important for bones and overall health.

The most common source of dietary calcium comes from dairy products, and without these, vegans are at risk of having lower calcium levels, which can put their bone health in danger.

### Omega-3s

Vegan diets do not include fish, eggs, or sea vegetables, which are the main sources of these healthy heart- and memory-protecting fats. There are plant-based fatty acids that can be converted to omega-3s, but not with any great efficiency. When tested, vegans tend to have lower blood concentrations of omega-3s. In a study published in the *American Journal of Clinical Nutrition,* researchers from the University of Oxford found that of 196 men, those who were vegan had the lowest levels of omega-3 fatty acids when compared to meat eaters.

### Protein

Animal protein contains all the essential amino acids our bodies need. Amino acids are key for muscle mass and bone health. Many vegans don't meet their protein requirements, which puts them at an increased risk of anemia and lowers their access to many of the nutrients already described.

## Too rigid and unsustainable

Interestingly, there are actually more ex-vegans than there are current vegans. In fact, 70 percent of those who've tried veganism end up quitting, according to a survey done by the Humane Research Council in 2015 (see the image on the following page). According to their study, in a cross-sectional survey of 11,400 men and women, nearly three-fourths of those who tried veganism ended up abandoning it. The numbers are even higher for vegetarians. The survey takers reported a variety of reasons, but one of the most common was that being a vegan or vegetarian made them feel conspicuous, and even those participants who were sticking with the nonmeat lifestyle said they felt like they stood out because of their diet choices. A vegan diet can be a difficult one to follow when you travel or are away from home. Options can be severely limited and can lead to you making poor health choices (fries, chips, and cookies do not a healthy diet make). While some people do work hard to get all their nutrients through diet and go to all lengths to plan, pack, and order healthy vegan meals, these folks are the exception.

You are almost completely Ready for Tiny and Ready for Full. You know now that you deserve to be Tiny, and you deserve to be Full. You've established the necessary mind-set to be the success you've always dreamed about. You know that having a Tiny Waist means both inner and outer beauty, that being Full means

## Comparison Chart:
## Current Vegetarians/Vegans to Former and Never Vegetarians/Vegans

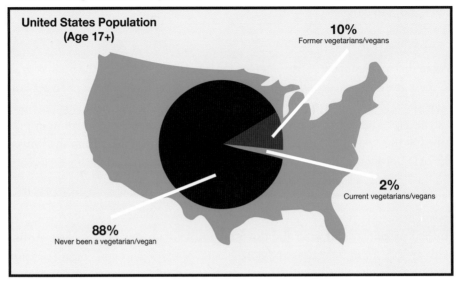

United States Population
(Age 17+)

10%
Former vegetarians/vegans

2%
Current vegetarians/vegans

88%
Never been a vegetarian/vegan

never feeling hungry or deprived, and that optimizing a vegan lifestyle is the key to being both Tiny and Full™.

We have just one last glitch to sort through—the vegan dilemma. The dilemma comes from the fact that although following a vegan lifestyle is beneficial in so many obvious ways, it's ultimately difficult to sustain and can be lacking essential nutrients. While you do increase fiber, vitamins, minerals, and antioxidants, and lower risks of many chronic diseases by eating vegan, not to mention the effortless path to slim living—it's hard to follow. So, what's the answer? Is there a way to get the best of both worlds? That's what I'm about to reveal to you. You know I wouldn't leave you hanging. You are just a page turn away from learning everything you need to know about how to incorporate everything positive about the vegan lifestyle, while leaving all the negatives behind in the dust. In the next chapter, we'll put all the pieces together, and you'll start taking the actions to get you going on becoming Tiny and Full™ forever. Turn the page to find out why deciding to Wake Up Vegan™ will transform your life!

# 3 Ready to Wake Up

41

So here we are. We've discussed getting Tiny and being Full for epic health; you've learned how to make the most of the calories you are going to eat by optimizing low-calorie-density foods; and you know all about the pros and cons of eating vegan. Now we've arrived at the time to put all the pieces together so that you can get started on the path to living a Tiny and Full™ life forever. Here's the plan:

1. Ready? First, we're going to discuss how setting the stage for success first thing in the morning will keep you strong all day long.

2. Set? Second, I'll teach you how you'll continue to eat healthy throughout the day to feel consistently Full, energized, and inspired—all while losing weight.

3. Go! Third, we'll get started. I'll walk you through how Tiny and Full™ will be working in your life on a daily basis.

Let's begin now.

# Wake Up Vegan™

When you start off your day by eating the most powerful, healing, and cleansing foods, you'll set the stage for success all day long. In Chapter 2, you learned how veganism is one of the healthiest and most healing diets available—for your body, and for the entire planet—all by relying on plant-based foods and reducing your intake of animal protein. Unfortunately, you also learned that veganism misses some vital nutrients that come from eating a more balanced diet and that the majority of people find that eating vegan is too rigid, limits options too drastically, and ultimately is not sustainable long term. Still, I want you to eat vegan. But that doesn't mean that you have to eat vegan all day long for the rest of your life. You can actually get all the benefits of a vegan lifestyle on a part-time basis. I'm going to teach you a realistic, satisfying, and fulfilling way of eating vegan that will allow you to get a Tiny Waist in 12 weeks and to continue eating for epic health and happiness for the rest of your life. You'll pump up your levels of all nutrients, you'll lower your calorie intake while always feeling Full, you'll slash your risk of chronic diseases, and you'll boost your levels of energy and immunity.

## The Wake Up Vegan™ solution

The solution is to Wake Up Vegan™! By following vegan eating principles each and every morning, you'll start your day off ahead of the game by nourishing your body with excellent sources of plant-based foods that are also naturally low in calorie density. You can eat satisfying and full plates, bowls, and cups of food that will lower your overall calories without you ever feeling hungry or deprived. Being a vegan in the morning is like giving yourself a daily detox. You'll cleanse your body each morning and then continue to eat a healthy balanced diet throughout the rest of the day. You really can optimize your health and happiness and be Tiny and Full™ by front-loading your morning with fruits and veggies. By Waking Up Vegan, you will also reap these other benefits:

- Enjoy younger-looking skin, stronger nails, and more luxurious hair

- Reduce the intensity of PMS symptoms

- Decrease body odor

- Boost your immunity

- Lose weight

- Lower your blood pressure

- Protect your eyesight

- Reduce your risk of heart disease, high cholesterol, diabetes, cancer, osteoporosis, obesity, and stroke

- Increase your energy

- Feel happier and more relaxed

- Help the planet by reducing greenhouse gases

By eating vegan in the morning and eating low-calorie-density foods all day long, you'll maximize your nutrient intake, feel Full all day, and reduce calories to get a Tiny Waist in 12 weeks!

## Morning is magical

You could eat vegan any time of the day, but there are a number of reasons, backed by research, that starting your day with a successful action such as eating vegan sets the stage for you to be successful all day long. Why? Morning is when your willpower is strongest.

Roy Baumeister, director of social psychology at Florida State University and author of *Willpower: Rediscovering the Greatest Human Strength,* has published numerous studies which show that determination and drive are almost always strongest in the morning hours when you are fresh. That's because willpower is like a muscle. It's strongest when it's been given adequate rest and restoration. Also like a muscle, as willpower is used as you go through the day, it becomes fatigued. What drains willpower is resisting trigger foods, making healthy decisions, dealing with difficult people, driving in traffic, being awake—basically just dealing with the normal demands of everyday life such as your work, partner, kids, your house, daily chores, and so on. That's why people tend to make healthier decisions in the morning, but by evening time, they are too tired to stick to healthy goals. Research shows that when your willpower is drained, you are more susceptible to overeating because the impulse control center in your brain becomes more vulnerable.

You can protect your willpower by Waking Up Vegan. According to Baumeister's research, the key is practicing healthy actions on a daily basis, such as starting off with the healthiest, most energizing, and most nourishing meal possible for breakfast. This strategy works both ways because you start off your day by consciously choosing foods that are good for you and because you set the tone for eating healthy, low-calorie-density foods all day long. You'll eat less while feeling Full. You'll have front-loaded your motivation muscle, and you'll strengthen your willpower to stave off temptations later in the day. It's an automated way to stay Full while eating the least amount of calories.

The other component of morning magic is that the physiological and biological chemical reactions of digesting breakfast help you stay Full throughout the day and lower your susceptibility to overeating later in the day. In one study, UK brain researchers from the Imperial College London used MRI scans to study the effects of

## Vegan Protein Powder

Vegans typically lack protein in their diets, and protein is an important part of breakfast because it helps keep you Full for longer than just fruits and vegetables. Research on breakfast shows that protein helps people to feel less hungry later in the day (people who eat just carbs for breakfast or skip breakfast tend to eat more calories throughout the day and more calories overall). While fruits and vegetables are highly nutritious, they are also quickly digested and can leave you craving more sustenance. Thankfully, I've discovered a fantastic solution to getting protein while sticking with vegan eating in the morning—pea protein powder. It's a relatively new addition to the protein powder family and is showing a lot of promise in the nutrition research community. Why go vegan for your protein? Let's count the ways:

- **It helps you stay Full:** Pea protein powder is made from isolating the protein in peas, so it's high in protein. At about 10–20 grams per scoop of powder, pea protein powder will keep you feeling Full and satisfied all morning long. In a study published in *Nutrition Journal,* researchers found that pea protein was just as satisfying as protein powder made with casein (made from milk protein) and more filling than protein powders made with whey and egg.

- **It's planet-friendly:** As discussed in the previous chapter, reducing your intake of animal protein is a great way to be more planet-friendly.

- **It's delicious:** Protein pea powder is delicious and comes in all the typical flavors—vanilla, chocolate, and unflavored. You can create delectable, creamy, frothy, fully satisfying, and fully vegan shakes.

skipping breakfast. The researchers found that the MRI scans of the people who ate breakfast didn't elicit dramatic brain changes when shown pictures of pizza, cake, or chocolate. However, when the researchers viewed the MRIs of the people who skipped their morning meal, they saw brains that lit up like a fireworks show on the 4th of July. The areas of the brain that were stimulated in the breakfast-skippers were the areas that control impulse, appetite, and cravings.

In Chapter 4, you'll find the Tiny and Full™ meal planners that provide you with a daily Wake Up Vegan™ breakfast plan complete with plenty of juicy fruits and savory vegetables, along with protein. It's important to include protein, especially if you are like me and have a hard time making it until lunch. Protein will help keep you Full and satisfied for the hours between meals. I've found a vegan protein pow-

- **It's gluten free:** If you are among the estimated 10 percent of people who struggle with gluten or grain intolerance, or if you've been diagnosed with celiac disease, pea protein powder is a great option for you. It's 100 percent gluten free.

- **It blends beautifully:** Many protein powders have a chalky, clumpy, or grainy texture or tendency. Not pea protein powder. It dissolves easily in water and blends into a creamy smooth shake. Even without a blender, pea protein powder blends easily in a shaker bottle.

- **It's hypoallergenic:** Many people have allergens to protein powders that contain whey, egg, soy, and casein (a milk protein). These ingredients can cause gas, bloating, and digestive discomfort. According to the Food Allergy Research & Education Organization, eight foods account for 90 percent of all allergic reactions: milk, eggs, peanuts, tree nuts, soy, wheat, fish, and shellfish. Peas are not among these. Pea protein powder is free of all allergens, making it the perfect choice.

There are many great pea protein powders on the market. I suggest one that is low in sugar and free of artificial additives. You can find my pea protein powder—made from incredible non-GMO, North American yellow peas and available in vanilla, chocolate, and plain flavors—at TinyandFull.com.

der that I love because it provides the 10g of satisfying protein you need while still allowing you to eat vegan in the morning (see the "Vegan Protein Powder," box on pages 60–61, for more information).

# All-Day Healthy Eating

Now that you know how to start your day off right, we can talk about how you'll keep eating healthy throughout the day to be Tiny and Full™. In the next section, you'll be given meal planners that will make eating the Tiny and Full™ way a no-brainer, but it's important for you to understand the logic behind this new way of eating. This will be especially helpful for those unavoidable occasions when you might be stuck without this book or a prepacked meal. I want you to always be prepared to keep your calorie density low and to never feel hungry or deprived.

Remember the Tiny and Full™ Levels Chart on pages 28–29? I suggest that you make a copy of that page and carry it in your pocket or purse. You can also take a picture with your smartphone or visit TinyandFull.com to get a digital copy. You can make sure to eat low-calorie-density foods all day by choosing the foods listed in Level 1 as often as possible, then use those foods in Levels 2 to 4 as condiments by dipping into Level 2 first, and using Level 3 more sparingly. Your Level 1 foods are your go-to foods for feeling satisfied on fewer calories. Here you'll find lots of vegetables and fruits, which are full of nutrients but with a very low calorie density. You'll already be ahead of the game by Waking Up Vegan, but it's a good idea to keep this trend going throughout your day. Try to minimize or avoid Level 4 as much as possible. Use Level 4 oils, such as olive oil, in moderation.

Next, read on for my favorite all-day healthy eating tips.

## Make meat a condiment

Use meat and animal products as condiments. The Western way of eating makes meat the star of the show, which means too many calories and often too many heart-clogging fats. Instead of ordering or grilling up a huge slab of steak, choose a lean cut, and slice it into small pieces. Build bigger meals by incorporating your side dishes and your protein together. Instead of having a small serving of vegetables on the side of your plate, stir-fry up a generous portion of vegetables, such as zucchini, red bell peppers, spinach, carrots, and snow peas, or mix up a large colorful salad of greens, peppers, tomatoes, carrots, shredded cabbage, and cucumbers, and top with chosen bits of protein. Your belly will be Full, but you'll stay way under your calorie quota.

## Soup equals satisfaction

When liquids are combined with solid food, your body treats it as a whole meal, says Barbara Rolls, author of *The Ultimate Volumetrics Diet*. This seems to trigger your brain to feel satisfied. Your eyes see a large portion, your senses of taste and smell are fed, and you feel Full. When Rolls serves soup in her lab, she sees her subjects shave 20 percent of the calories off the meal that follows. There is an enormous body of research on soup and weight loss that began back in the 1980s. These studies consistently find that when people eat soup, they cut calories—up to four times as much as people who don't include this liquid food in their diets. For reasons not fully understood, drinking water separately doesn't provide the same satiating effects as eating it mixed in with food to make a soup.

## Go big

When you are making your lunches and dinners, think large in terms of size, but low in terms of calories. Make a plentiful plate or container of salad, a big bowl of soup, or a generous dish of stir-fried vegetables. By using a foundation of vegetables and water (in soups), you'll create satisfying meals that will stay well within your calorie range.

## Prep your fruits and veggies

Make sure to keep a container of clean veggies such as sliced cucumbers, baby carrots, sugar snap peas, celery sticks, or grape tomatoes for quick low-calorie-density snacking. Ditto on the fruits—I love to keep a bowl of strawberries, cubed melon, or grapes always in my fridge for quick snacking.

## Rate your hunger

Remember to use the 1 to 10 hunger rating scale on page 26 from Chapter 2. Starting today, pay attention to how you feel. Start listening to the signals your body gives you about feeling hungry. How do you feel right now? Is your stomach growling or aching? Do you feel pleasantly Full? Before eating your next meal or snack, ask yourself, "Am I hungry right now?" After putting this query to yourself, use the scale to rate your hunger, with 1 being starving, and 10 being so stuffed you can't move. Don't stop there. As you eat your meal, pause and check in again, asking, "Am I still hungry?" When your rating reaches a 4 or 5, it's time to stop. If you aren't sure, put down your utensils, wait for five minutes or so, and then ask yourself again if you're hungry. Stay conscious throughout your entire meal. It may help to keep your eating area quiet and without distractions from a television or computer. It might even help to eat a meal or two in solitude. Over time, you will naturally begin to recognize your healthy hunger and full signals.

# How to Get Started

Before you turn to the next section and start following the meal plans, it's important to do some prep work and then continue to track your progress in several different ways. Below you'll find directions on how to set a baseline for yourself, your weight, and your waist and hips, as well as how to track your progress daily and weekly to keep your motivation optimally revved.

But first, let me summarize the steps to getting started:

Take a weekly selfie.

Weigh yourself daily.

Choose your calorie goal.

Take a weekly measurement of your waist and hips.

Write down your accountability partners.

Join me socially.

Sign the Success Contract.

## Take a weekly selfie

During the next 12 weeks, you'll be taking pictures once a week to track your progress. You'll also track your weight, but it's important to follow the progress you see in your photos. There are many changes you'll be able to detect in your photos that a scale won't show you. This is especially important when you want to lose a moderate or small amount of weight. Without visible evidence of your body's changes, you won't be able to notice the subtle improvements that can be seen in a picture. Here's how to take your selfie:

- Set a reminder on your phone and/or computer calendar so you'll have an automated alarm that triggers you to take your picture.

- Always shoot your picture at the same time of the day and on the same day of the week. I recommend taking your photo first thing in the morning, before you have breakfast.

- Wear the same clothes for each picture. I recommend something form fitting, or, even better, wear a bikini, bathing suit, or a bra and underwear.

- Take your photo in the same location, same background, and same lighting.

- Make sure your photo captures your entire body.

- Take two pictures. Take one picture with you facing front and another shot that captures your profile (a side view).

- Stand in the same posture, with your feet together, and your hands slightly away from your sides.

- Don't pose. Don't suck in your belly or try to hide your thighs. Stand in a relaxed manner.

## Weigh yourself daily

It used to be that you were only supposed to weigh yourself once a week, but no more. Today's nutritionists will tell you, and I agree, that you can keep your motivation at its highest by stepping on the scale once each morning. According to a recent study published in the *Journal of the Academy of Nutrition and Dietetics,* weighing yourself every day boosts motivation and leads to greater weight loss. For the study, researchers asked 91 men and women, ages 18 to 60, to either weigh themselves daily or to weigh themselves once a week. At the end of six months, the daily weighers lost 13 to 14 pounds, while the weekly weighers lost about 7 pounds. These daily scale-steppers also reduced the calories they consumed each day, increased their exercise, and reduced their television-viewing time more than those who weighed themselves less often. Still not convinced? In another study, University of Minnesota researchers tracked the weighing habits of 1,800 men and women who were trying to lose weight. The researchers found that those who did a daily weigh-in lost an average of 12 pounds over two years, while those who weighed weekly lost only 6 pounds. Not only did the daily weight watchers lose twice as much weight, they were less likely to regain the weight lost.

### How to track your weight

First choose a goal weight that is healthy and realistic. Take a moment to think about the history of your weight gains and losses over the past years. What was your lowest weight ever? Where does your weight seem to settle when you are taking action to be your healthiest ever? If you feel daunted by the amount of weight you have to lose, focus on reducing your weight by 10 percent to start. If you weigh 180, you'll focus on losing 18 pounds. Then, when you reach 162, you'll lose 16 pounds, and so on. In this way, your weight loss will feel more attainable, and you'll stay more motivated. Plus, setting up mini-achievements will give you more opportunities to reward yourself—another great way to stay motivated!

*Baseline weight*

Tomorrow morning, as soon as you wake up, step on the scale and write your baseline weight in the space below:

**Baseline Weight** _____ .

*Daily weight*

Each morning from now until day 84, repeat your scale-stepping action first thing in the morning and write your weight in the provided tracker on page 56. Don't fret if you see some fluctuations. Your weight can go up a pound or two based on retained liquid, sodium, or due to your menstrual cycle, but as long as you follow the Tiny and Full™ menus and meal planners, you'll steadily lose one to two pounds a week.

## Choose your calorie goal

Based on your weight, choose your calorie level. In the next section of the book, you'll begin your menus and meal planners. You select your calorie level based on your current weight. You may need to adjust your calorie level as you lose weight. Please refer to the following chart.

| Current Weight | Women:<br>Calories Per Day | Men:<br>Calories Per Day |
| --- | --- | --- |
| Less than 150 lbs | 1,200 | 1,400 |
| 150–199 | 1,400 | 1,600 |
| 200–249 | 1,600 | 1,800 |
| 250–299 | 2,000 | 2,000 |
| More than 300 lbs | For every 50 lbs. over 300, add 100 additional calories per day | For every 50 lbs. over 300, add 100 additional calories per day |

## Take a weekly measurement of your waist and hips

In Chapter 1, we discussed the importance of measuring your waist and keeping track of your waist-to-hip ratio. As a quick review, your waist-to-hip ratio is the measurement that shows the size of your waist in relation to your hips. A healthy waist-to-hip ratio for women is 0.7, and for men, it's 1.0. To take this measurement, take a fabric tape measure and, while sucking in your belly, measure your waist at the level of your belly button. Next, measure your hips at the largest point around your bottom. Finally, divide your waist size by your hip size. For example, if you have hips that are 46 inches and a waist that is 40 inches, then your waist-to-hip ratio is 0.86. Write all three measurements in the appropriate spaces in the tracker that starts on page 56. Seeing the inches melt off your body is a great way to stay motivated. Plus, a healthy waist circumference—35 inches for women, 40 inches for men—has been linked to better health as well. The Nurses' Health Study, one of the largest and longest studies to date that measures abdominal obesity, found that after 16 years, women who have the largest waist circumferences had nearly double the risk for dying from heart disease, an increased risk of dying from cancer, and an increased risk of dying from any cause, compared to women with the lowest waist circumferences.

## Write down your accountability partners

I want you to bring all the pieces together by creating your own team of support, by signing the following Success Contract, and by committing to checking in with me on the social media sites I'm including below. To ensure your success, make a commitment to yourself, track your weight and waist measurements, take those selfies, and enlist a group of friends (me included!) and family to support your efforts.

Your group of cheerleaders can include family members, coworkers, and good friends—anyone you feel comfortable communicating with openly and honestly. People in your inner support team must be caring and nonjudgmental, and they must be willing to listen to you and support you. Start by thinking of three people you'd like to invite into your inner support team. List their names (just their names for now) in the blanks on the left below:

Name and Contact Info: _____     Text Contact: _____

Name and Contact Info: _____     Phone Contact: _____

Name and Contact Info: _____     Accountability Contact: _____

Now I want you to appoint each person a contact category and write it in the blank space above, along with his or her contact information.

Here are the types of contact categories to choose from:

- Text contact: Designate one of the three people you listed as your texting contact, and fill in her cell phone number in the contact information area. Anytime you feel that you need to reach out for encouragement, shoot a text to this person and tell her how you're feeling. Feel free to designate more than one person to this category. Invite friends and family who may want to lose weight to lose to join you on this journey.

- Phone contact: In the second space, list a friend or family member as a phone buddy, and fill in his home, work, and cell phone numbers. This buddy will help you when you need immediate support.

- Accountability contact: The last person on your inner support team is your accountability contact. This person will help you stay accountable for your weight-loss goal by talking to you for up to 15 minutes every night during your first week, preferably at the end of each day.

## Join me socially

Please join the Tiny and Full™ community to share with me and with others following the Tiny and Full™ path to epic health and happiness. You'll find motivational tools and community support, and you'll also be able to cheer others on in their weight-loss journeys. Join me at these social media sites to post your photos and share your journey of success:

- Facebook.com/TinyandFull

- Instagram.com/TinyandFull

- Twitter.com/TinyandFull

- TinyandFull.com

- #TinyandFull

## Sign the Success Contract

Please read the short commitment contract on the next page. I encourage you to rewrite this in your own hand. Feel free to personalize this Success Contract, adding any details that will help remind you of your internal motivation for wanting to change your life for the better. Use this written oath as a reminder to yourself that you are making YOU a priority. I know you want to look and feel healthy, but you've got to lay the mental foundation first. Think about the journey you are about to embark on. Do you want this? There are going to be good days, and, I won't lie,

# The Success Contract

I, _____

commit to following the Tiny and Full™ menus and principles

for the next 12 weeks, starting on _____,

because I am worth it. I know that I deserve to be Tiny and

Full™. By tracking my progress in photos, weighing myself daily,

and measuring my waist weekly, I am committing to loving

myself, my body, and my life. By signing my name below, I am

acknowledging that I deserve radiance, energy, health, and

vitality. I promise myself to live in accordance with the rules of

Tiny and Full™. By following the eating plan to the letter, I am

creating what I deserve—epic health and happiness. I deserve a

Full Life. So be it.

Sign _____

Date _____

you will have some days where you'll struggle. Life will keep coming with all its ups and downs, no matter what you decide to do for yourself. You will be better armed with this book and all the powerful Tiny and Full™ tools in your back pocket, but ultimately *you* are the key. You must believe in yourself, believe that you can do this, and believe that you deserve a better life, better health, and more happiness. I already know that you deserve all of this—but you have to do your part by signing the following contract. This document that you'll write and sign is nonnegotiable, binding, and permanent. After you sign this commitment contract, there's no going back. You are promising to live your best life ever, to feed yourself only the best foods, and to treat your body with the utmost respect.

## Selfie, Weight, Waist Tracker

Track the weekly and daily dates of your progress photos, your weight, and your shrinking waist and hips all in one place. Jot the date for your selfie and print it out. I encourage you to buy a small photo book to save your selfies in, or better yet, tape them in your bedroom where you can see them to keep your motivation strong. Later in this chapter, you'll find weekly spots for your selfie date, waist measurement, hip measurement, and hip-to-waist ratio as well as, and weekly and daily spots for your weight. Use the tracker so you can easily watch your progress improving over the next 12 weeks. You'll keep your drive and determination high by being able to see all your progress in one place. Be sure to pause as the weeks pass by to review each of the previous weeks. By taking notice of the inches and pounds that melt off your body, you'll create a natural reward. It's true: research shows that just pausing to take notice of positive experiences will stimulate the reward centers of your brain, which will inherently drive you to keep making healthy choices.

Feel free to jot notes in the white spaces on the following pages. It's a great opportunity to take notice of positive changes. Write down what works for you in the coming weeks, record circumstances where you successfully overcome obstacles and stick to your Tiny and Full™ plan, and be sure to take note as your clothes get roomier and as tasks such as carrying groceries or running up the stairs gets easier. It all counts—and the more you write, the more you remember.

Congratulations! You've done all the prep work necessary to get started. You now know how to Wake Up Vegan™ to jump-start your day and to set the stage for getting your Tiny Waist and feeling Full all day. You've learned the strategies you need to plan healthy eating that will keep you satisfied and Full, never ravenous or deprived. You've created a team of support and signed a contract of commitment. You've taken the time to track your weight, waist, hips, waist-to-hip ratio, and your progress photos. With this strong foundation, you can't fail!

In the next chapter, you'll find detailed meal planners that I've created for you. Here you'll get a plan so automated that you can save all your brainpower for staying positive and powerful. And, if you ever find yourself stuck without your planners, you can easily stay on the Tiny and Full™ plan by remembering the following rules:

1. Keep calorie density low.

2. Eat vegan in the morning.

3. Keep all meals to 300 calories.

4. Keep all snacks to 100 calories, unless you fall into a higher calorie level.

5. Stay within your personalized calorie allotment.

That's it. You're now ready to get started. You've got this. It's simple. Fruits and veggies are your go-to friends. All your foods fall into a level, and it's always easy to find the calorie density of a given food by taking calories per serving and dividing by grams per serving (refer to page 25 in Chapter 2).

## Week 1

**Day 1:**

| Selfie | Waist | Hips | Waist-to-Hip Ratio | Weight |
|--------|-------|------|--------------------|--------|
|        |       |      |                    |        |

**Day 2:**                    Weight:

**Day 3:**                    Weight:

**Day 4:**                    Weight:

**Day 5:**                    Weight:

**Day 6:**                    Weight:

**Day 7:**                    Weight:

## Week 2

**Day 8:**

| Selfie | Waist | Hips | Waist-to-Hip Ratio | Weight |
|--------|-------|------|--------------------|--------|
|        |       |      |                    |        |

**Day 9:**                    Weight:

**Day 10:**                   Weight:

**Day 11:**                   Weight:

**Day 12:**                   Weight:

**Day 13:**                   Weight:

**Day 14:**                   Weight:

# Week 3

**Day 15:**

| Selfie | Waist | Hips | Waist-to-Hip Ratio | Weight |
|--------|-------|------|--------------------|--------|
|        |       |      |                    |        |

**Day 16:**          Weight:

**Day 17:**          Weight:

**Day 18:**          Weight:

**Day 19:**          Weight:

**Day 20:**          Weight:

**Day 21:**          Weight:

# Week 4

**Day 22:**

| Selfie | Waist | Hips | Waist-to-Hip Ratio | Weight |
|--------|-------|------|--------------------|--------|
|        |       |      |                    |        |

**Day 23:**          Weight:

**Day 24:**          Weight:

**Day 25:**          Weight:

**Day 26:**          Weight:

**Day 27:**          Weight:

**Day 28:**          Weight:

## Week 5

**Day 29:**

| Selfie | Waist | Hips | Waist-to-Hip Ratio | Weight |
|--------|-------|------|--------------------|--------|
|        |       |      |                    |        |

**Day 30:**                  Weight:

**Day 31:**                  Weight:

**Day 32:**                  Weight:

**Day 33:**                  Weight:

**Day 34:**                  Weight:

**Day 35:**                  Weight:

## Week 6

**Day 36:**

| Selfie | Waist | Hips | Waist-to-Hip Ratio | Weight |
|--------|-------|------|--------------------|--------|
|        |       |      |                    |        |

**Day 37:**                  Weight:

**Day 38:**                  Weight:

**Day 39:**                  Weight:

**Day 40:**                  Weight:

**Day 41:**                  Weight:

**Day 42:**                  Weight:

## Week 7

**Day 43:**

| Selfie | Waist | Hips | Waist-to-Hip Ratio | Weight |
|--------|-------|------|--------------------|--------|
|        |       |      |                    |        |

**Day 44:**          **Weight:**

**Day 45:**          **Weight:**

**Day 46:**          **Weight:**

**Day 47:**          **Weight:**

**Day 48:**          **Weight:**

**Day 49:**          **Weight:**

## Week 8

**Day 50:**

| Selfie | Waist | Hips | Waist-to-Hip Ratio | Weight |
|--------|-------|------|--------------------|--------|
|        |       |      |                    |        |

**Day 51:**          **Weight:**

**Day 52:**          **Weight:**

**Day 53:**          **Weight:**

**Day 54:**          **Weight:**

**Day 55:**          **Weight:**

**Day 56:**          **Weight:**

## Week 9

**Day 57:**

| Selfie | Waist | Hips | Waist-to-Hip Ratio | Weight |
|--------|-------|------|--------------------|--------|
|        |       |      |                    |        |

**Day 58:** Weight:

**Day 59:** Weight:

**Day 60:** Weight:

**Day 61:** Weight:

**Day 62:** Weight:

**Day 63:** Weight:

## Week 10

**Day 64:**

| Selfie | Waist | Hips | Waist-to-Hip Ratio | Weight |
|--------|-------|------|--------------------|--------|
|        |       |      |                    |        |

**Day 65:** Weight:

**Day 66:** Weight:

**Day 67:** Weight:

**Day 68:** Weight:

**Day 69:** Weight:

**Day 70:** Weight:

## Week 11

**Day 71:**

| Selfie | Waist | Hips | Waist-to-Hip Ratio | Weight |
|--------|-------|------|--------------------|--------|
|        |       |      |                    |        |

**Day 72:**              Weight:

**Day 73:**              Weight:

**Day 74:**              Weight:

**Day 75:**              Weight:

**Day 76:**              Weight:

**Day 77:**              Weight:

## Week 12

**Day 78:**

| Selfie | Waist | Hips | Waist-to-Hip Ratio | Weight |
|--------|-------|------|--------------------|--------|
|        |       |      |                    |        |

**Day 79:**              Weight:

**Day 80:**              Weight:

**Day 81:**              Weight:

**Day 82:**              Weight:

**Day 83:**              Weight:

**Day 84:**              Weight:

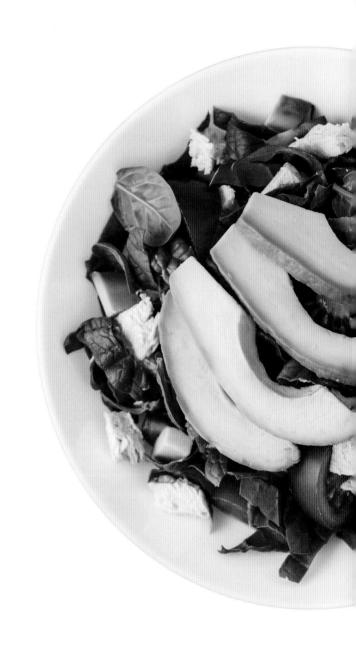

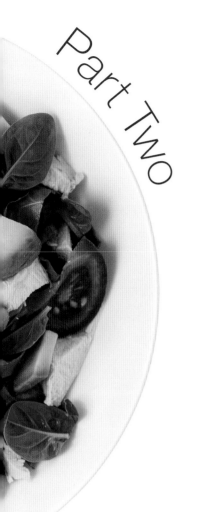

# Part Two

# How to Be Tiny and Full™

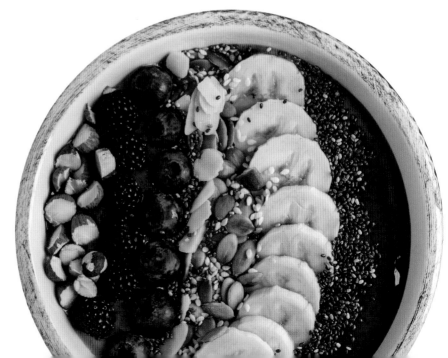

# 4 Your 12-Week Meal Planners

Now that you understand how Tiny and Full™ works, it's time to get started! I have provided you with a 12-week eating plan to guide you toward the types of food you should eat. Over the years, my clients have said that they like to have a consistent meal planner to follow so there are no surprises. Here you have my best strategy in four unique meal planners that repeat throughout the 12 weeks.

The meal planners all start at 1,200 calories with three main meals—breakfast, lunch, and dinner—and include snacks and treats. The meals are all around 300 calories, and the snacks and treats are around 100 calories.

If your calorie goal is higher than 1,200 calories, you can increase the portions of your meals or increase your snacks. If you find you aren't losing weight or you're losing weight too quickly, adjust your caloric intake accordingly to find the right balance for you.

You'll notice that the meal planners include some of the recipes from Chapters 8–10, as well as some quick, toss-together meals. I recommend not making any substitutions to the meal planners to ensure your success. However, if you do decide to make substitutions, keep an eye out for the calories and adjust accordingly.

Let's eat!

## When You're in a Pinch

On-the-go? In a pinch? I get it, I've been there. In fact, I'm probably there right now! I travel a lot for work, and even when I'm home, I'm running around with my kids or dashing off to the office. If you're constantly on the run as well, my go-to option is the Tiny and Full™ Fiber Bar (you can find these at TinyandFull.com).

Do you have any Tiny and Full™ on-the-go options you like? Tag @TinyandFull or use #TinyandFull on Instagram to share with me.

## Day 1

### Breakfast

2 slices vegan whole-wheat toast topped with 1 tbsp. almond butter and ¼ cup halved strawberries (312 calories)

### Snack

¾ cup grapes (78 calories)

390 calories

### Lunch

Organic Chicken Caesar Salad (page 212) (310 calories)

### Snack

6 oz. plain Greek yogurt with 3 sliced strawberries (112 calories)

422 calories

### Dinner

3 oz. cooked wild salmon, ½ cup whole-grain brown rice, 1 cup sautéed kale, salt and pepper to taste (287 calories)

287 calories

### Treat

Banana Berry Ice Cream (page 255) (96 calories)

96 calories

**1,195 Total Calories**

## Day 2

### Breakfast

Tropical Mango Blast (page 169) (243 calories)

### Snack

1 orange with ½ cup blueberries (104 calories)

347 calories

### Lunch

Tomato Gazpacho Fresca (page 215) with 2 slices whole-wheat toast (346 calories)

### Snack

10 celery sticks with 1 tbsp. peanut butter (100 calories)

446 calories

### Dinner

Guilt-Free Zucchini Pasta (page 246) (222 calories)

222 calories

### Treat

6 oz. plain Greek yogurt mixed with cinnamon (100 calories)

100 calories

**1,115 Total Calories**

## Day 3

### Breakfast

2 slices vegan whole-wheat toast topped with 1 tbsp. almond butter and ¼ cup halved strawberries (312 calories)

### Snack

¾ cup grapes (78 calories)

390 calories

### Lunch

2 cups spinach tossed with 2 chopped hard-boiled eggs, ½ cup chopped red bell pepper, ½ cup sliced white mushrooms, ¼ cup avocado slices, and 2 tbsp. balsamic vinegar (283 calories)

### Snack

6 oz. plain Greek yogurt with 3 sliced strawberries (112 calories)

395 calories

### Dinner

California Fish Tacos (page 227) (251 calories)

251 calories

### Treat

Banana Berry Ice Cream (page 255) (96 calories)

96 calories

**1,132 Total Calories**

## Day 4

### Breakfast

Tropical Mango Blast (page 169) (243 calories)

### Snack

1 orange with ½ cup blueberries (104 calories)

347 calories

### Lunch

Organic Chicken Caesar Salad (page 212) (310 calories)

### Snack

10 celery sticks with 1 tbsp. peanut butter (100 calories)

410 calories

### Dinner

3 oz. cooked wild salmon, ½ cup whole-grain brown rice, 1 cup sautéed kale, salt and pepper to taste (287 calories)

287 calories

### Treat

6 oz. plain Greek yogurt mixed with cinnamon (100 calories)

100 calories

**1,144 Total Calories**

## Day 5

### Breakfast

2 slices vegan whole-wheat toast topped with 1 tbsp. almond butter and ¼ cup halved strawberries (312 calories)

### Snack

¾ cup grapes (78 calories)

390 calories

### Lunch

Tomato Gazpacho Fresca (page 215) with 2 slices whole-wheat toast (346 calories)

### Snack

6 oz. plain Greek yogurt with 3 sliced strawberries (112 calories)

458 calories

### Dinner

Guilt-Free Zucchini Pasta (page 246) (222 calories)

222 calories

### Treat

Banana Berry Ice Cream (page 255) (96 calories)

96 calories

**1,166 Total Calories**

## Day 6

### Breakfast

Tropical Mango Blast (page 169) (243 calories)

### Snack

1 orange with ½ cup blueberries (104 calories)

347 calories

### Lunch

2 cups spinach tossed with 2 chopped hard-boiled eggs, ½ cup chopped red bell pepper, ½ cup sliced white mushrooms, ¼ cup avocado slices, and 2 tbsp. balsamic vinegar (283 calories)

### Snack

10 celery sticks with 1 tbsp. peanut butter (100 calories)

383 calories

### Dinner

California Fish Tacos (page 227) (251 calories)

251 calories

### Treat

6 oz. plain Greek yogurt mixed with cinnamon (100 calories)

100 calories

**1,081 Total Calories**

## Week 1

### Day 7

**Breakfast**

2 slices vegan whole-wheat toast topped with 1 tbsp. almond butter and ¼ cup halved strawberries (312 calories)

**Snack**

¾ cup grapes (78 calories)

390 calories

**Lunch**

Organic Chicken Caesar Salad (page 212) (310 calories)

**Snack**

6 oz. plain Greek yogurt with 3 sliced strawberries (112 calories)

422 calories

**Dinner**

3 oz. cooked wild salmon, ½ cup whole-grain brown rice, 1 cup sautéed kale, salt and pepper to taste (287 calories)

287 calories

**Treat**

Banana Berry Ice Cream (page 255) (96 calories)

96 calories

**1,195 Total Calories**

## Week 2

### Day 8

**Breakfast**

Sunshine Cinnamon Nut Quinoa (page 189) (274 calories)

**Snack**

1 small banana (90 calories)

364 calories

**Lunch**

In a medium bowl, toss together ½ cup watermelon, ½ cup chopped cucumber, ¼ cup chopped avocado, and ¼ cup chopped radishes with 1 tsp. olive oil. Sprinkle with salt and pepper to taste. Serve with ½ cup Greek yogurt drizzled in 1 tsp. olive oil and salt and pepper. (243 calories)

**Snack**

15 baby carrots with 2 tbsp. tzatziki (83 calories)

326 calories

**Dinner**

Grilled Tilapia Grapefruit Salad (page 237) (260 calories)

260 calories

**Treat**

Cocoa Bean Brownie (page 256) (112 calories)

112 calories

**1,062 Total Calories**

## Day 9

### Breakfast

1 grapefruit with 1 slice vegan whole-wheat toast topped with 1 tbsp. almond butter (241 calories)

### Snack

1 medium apple (95 calories)

336 calories

### Lunch

Sweet Arugula Pear Salad (page 216) with 1 slice whole-grain toast (310 calories)

### Snack

1 cup blueberries (85 calories)

395 calories

### Dinner

3 oz. roasted chicken with 2 cups roasted vegetables and ½ baked sweet potato (272 calories)

272 calories

### Treat

2 tbsp. light whipped cream topped with 1 cup sliced strawberries and ¼ sliced banana (90 calories)

90 calories

**1,093 Total Calories**

## Day 10

### Breakfast

Sunshine Cinnamon Nut Quinoa (page 189) (274 calories)

### Snack

1 small banana (90 calories)

364 calories

### Lunch

Garden Greek Salad (page 245) (312 calories)

### Snack

15 baby carrots with 2 tbsp. tzatziki (83 calories)

395 calories

### Dinner

Spaghetti Squash Pasta (page 250) (300 calories)

300 calories

### Treat

Cocoa Bean Brownie (page 256) (112 calories)

112 calories

**1,171 Total Calories**

## Day 11

### Breakfast

1 grapefruit with 1 slice vegan whole-wheat toast topped with 1 tbsp. almond butter (241 calories)

### Snack

1 medium apple (95 calories)

336 calories

### Lunch

In a medium bowl, toss together ½ cup watermelon, ½ cup chopped cucumber, ¼ cup chopped avocado, and ¼ cup chopped radishes with 1 tsp. olive oil. Sprinkle with salt and pepper to taste. Serve with ½ cup Greek yogurt drizzled in 1 tsp. olive oil and salt and pepper. (243 calories)

### Snack

1 cup blueberries (85 calories)

328 calories

### Dinner

Grilled Tilapia Grapefruit Salad (page 237) (260 calories)

260 calories

### Treat

2 tbsp. light whipped cream topped with 1 cup sliced strawberries and ¼ sliced banana (90 calories)

90 calories

**1,014 Total Calories**

## Day 12

### Breakfast

Sunshine Cinnamon Nut Quinoa (page 189) (274 calories)

### Snack

1 small banana (90 calories)

364 calories

### Lunch

Sweet Arugula Pear Salad (page 216) with 1 slice whole-grain toast (310 calories)

### Snack

15 baby carrots with 2 tbsp. tzatziki (83 calories)

393 calories

### Dinner

3 oz. roasted chicken with 2 cups roasted vegetables and ½ baked sweet potato (272 calories)

272 calories

### Treat

Cocoa Bean Brownie (page 256) (112 calories)

112 calories

**1,141 Total Calories**

## Day 13

### Breakfast

1 grapefruit with 1 slice vegan whole-wheat toast topped with 1 tbsp. almond butter (241 calories)

### Snack

1 medium apple (95 calories)

336 calories

### Lunch

Garden Greek Salad (page 245) (312 calories)

### Snack

1 cup blueberries (85 calories)

397 calories

### Dinner

Spaghetti Squash Pasta (page 250) (300 calories)

300 calories

### Treat

2 tbsp. light whipped cream topped with 1 cup sliced strawberries and ¼ sliced banana (90 calories)

90 calories

**1,123 Total Calories**

## Day 14

### Breakfast

Sunshine Cinnamon Nut Quinoa (page 189) (274 calories)

### Snack

1 small banana (90 calories)

364 calories

### Lunch

In a medium bowl, toss together ½ cup watermelon, ½ cup chopped cucumber, ¼ cup chopped avocado, and ¼ cup chopped radishes with 1 tsp. olive oil. Sprinkle with salt and pepper to taste. Serve with ½ cup Greek yogurt drizzled in 1 tsp. olive oil and salt and pepper. (243 calories)

### Snack

15 baby carrots with 2 tbsp. tzatziki (83 calories)

326 calories

### Dinner

Grilled Tilapia Grapefruit Salad (page 237) (260 calories)

260 calories

### Treat

Cocoa Bean Brownie (page 256) (112 calories)

112 calories

**1,062 Total Calories**

## Day 15

### Breakfast

½ cup rolled oats with ½ cup raspberries and 1 cup unsweetened almond milk (252 calories)

### Snack

1 cup unsweetened applesauce sprinkled with cinnamon (100 calories)

352 calories

### Lunch

Turkocado Salad (page 219) (238 calories)

### Snack

1 cup cherries (95 calories)

333 calories

### Dinner

Baked Cauliflower Casserole (page 241) (250 calories)

250 calories

### Treat

2 slices Watermelon Lover's Pizza (page 272) with 3 oz. plain Greek yogurt (102 calories)

102 calories

**1,037 Total Calories**

## Day 16

### Breakfast

Sweet Greens Smoothie Bowl (page 181) (341 calories)

### Snack

4 medium strawberries dipped in 1 tbsp. melted dark chocolate (100 calories)

441 calories

### Lunch

1 small whole-wheat roll filled with 2 oz. grilled chicken, 1 leaf romaine lettuce, 1 slice tomato, and 1 tsp. mustard (276 calories)

### Snack

6 oz. plain Greek yogurt topped with 3 raspberries (103 calories)

379 calories

### Dinner

Sunshine Summer Salad (page 224) (289 calories)

289 calories

### Treat

1 medium frozen banana pureed into ice cream (105 calories)

105 calories

**1,214 Total Calories**

## Day 17

### Breakfast

½ cup rolled oats with ½ cup raspberries and 1 cup unsweetened almond milk (252 calories)

### Snack

1 cup unsweetened applesauce sprinkled with cinnamon (100 calories)

352 calories

### Lunch

Organic Artichoke Tomato Soup (page 249) (200 calories)

### Snack

1 cup cherries (95 calories)

295 calories

### Dinner

3 oz. roasted turkey breast, ½ cup sautéed mushrooms, ½ cup whole-grain brown rice, 1 pat butter (286 calories)

286 calories

### Treat

2 slices Watermelon Lover's Pizza (page 272) with 3 oz. plain Greek yogurt (102 calories)

102 calories

**1,035 Total Calories**

## Day 18

### Breakfast

Sweet Greens Smoothie Bowl (page 181) (341 calories)

### Snack

4 medium strawberries dipped in 1 tbsp. melted dark chocolate (100 calories)

441 calories

### Lunch

Turkocado Salad (page 219) (238 calories)

### Snack

6 oz. plain Greek yogurt topped with 3 raspberries (103 calories)

341 calories

### Dinner

Baked Cauliflower Casserole (page 241) (250 calories)

250 calories

### Treat

1 medium frozen banana pureed into ice cream (105 calories)

105 calories

**1,137 Total Calories**

## Day 19

### Breakfast

½ cup rolled oats with ½ cup raspberries and 1 cup unsweetened almond milk (252 calories)

### Snack

1 cup unsweetened applesauce sprinkled with cinnamon (100 calories)

352 calories

### Lunch

1 small whole-wheat roll filled with 2 oz. grilled chicken, 1 leaf romaine lettuce, 1 slice tomato, and 1 tsp. mustard (276 calories)

### Snack

1 cup cherries (95 calories)

371 calories

### Dinner

Sunshine Summer Salad (page 224) (289 calories)

289 calories

### Treat

2 slices Watermelon Lover's Pizza (page 272) with 3 oz. plain Greek yogurt (102 calories)

102 calories

**1,114 Total Calories**

## Day 20

### Breakfast

Sweet Greens Smoothie Bowl (page 181) (341 calories)

### Snack

4 medium strawberries dipped in 1 tbsp. melted dark chocolate (100 calories)

441 calories

### Lunch

Organic Artichoke Tomato Soup (page 249) (200 calories)

### Snack

6 oz. plain Greek yogurt topped with 3 raspberries (103 calories)

303 calories

### Dinner

3 oz. roasted turkey breast, ½ cup sautéed mushrooms, ½ cup whole-grain brown rice, 1 pat butter (286 calories)

286 calories

### Treat

1 medium frozen banana pureed into ice cream (105 calories)

105 calories

**1,135 Total Calories**

## Week 3

## Day 21

### Breakfast

½ cup rolled oats with ½ cup raspberries and 1 cup unsweetened almond milk (252 calories)

### Snack

1 cup unsweetened applesauce sprinkled with cinnamon (100 calories)

352 calories

### Lunch

Turkocado Salad (page 219) (238 calories)

### Snack

1 cup cherries (95 calories)

333 calories

### Dinner

Baked Cauliflower Casserole (page 241) (250 calories)

250 calories

### Treat

2 slices Watermelon Lover's Pizza (page 272) with 3 oz. plain Greek yogurt (102 calories)

250 calories

**1,037 Total Calories**

## Week 4

## Day 22

### Breakfast

Berry Blaster Bowl (page 177) (273 calories)

### Snack

1 medium apple (95 calories)

368 calories

### Lunch

2 slices whole-grain bread spread with 2 tbsp. hummus and topped with 4 (¼ inch) round cucumber slices, ½ small sliced red bell pepper, and ¼ cup baby spinach (290 calories)

### Snack

4 tbsp. wasabi peas (90 calories)

380 calories

### Dinner

Asparagus Cauliflower Pizza (page 238) (331 calories)

331 calories

### Treat

3 tbsp. whipped cream topped with ¼ cup blueberries and ½ cup sliced strawberries (81 calories)

81 calories

**1,160 Total Calories**

## Day 23

### Breakfast

2 slices vegan whole-wheat toast topped with 1 tbsp. peanut butter and ¼ cup sliced banana (247 calories)

### Snack

1 cup mixed berries tossed with 1 tbsp. lemon juice (100 calories)

347 calories

### Lunch

Strawberry Feta Summer Salad (page 211) with 1 slice whole-grain toast with butter (302 calories)

### Snack

1 orange with ½ cup blueberries (104 calories)

406 calories

### Dinner

Pan-Seared Salmon Salad (page 231) with ¼ cup whole-grain brown rice (273 calories)

273 calories

### Treat

2 Strawberry Yogurt Ice Pops (page 267) (100 calories)

100 calories

**1,126 Total Calories**

## Day 24

### Breakfast

Berry Blaster Bowl (page 177) (273 calories)

### Snack

1 medium apple (95 calories)

368 calories

### Lunch

Sunshine Summer Salad (page 224) (289 calories)

### Snack

4 tbsp. wasabi peas (90 calories)

379 calories

### Dinner

1 cup cooked whole-wheat pasta shells tossed with 1 cup arugula, 2 tbsp. shredded Romano cheese, ¼ cup cherry tomatoes, ½ tbsp. olive oil, and a dash of red pepper flakes (311 calories)

311 calories

### Treat

3 tbsp. whipped cream topped with ¼ cup blueberries and ½ cup sliced strawberries (81 calories)

81 calories

**1,139 Total Calories**

## Day 25

### Breakfast

2 slices vegan whole-wheat toast topped with 1 tbsp. peanut butter and ¼ cup sliced banana (247 calories)

### Snack

1 cup mixed berries tossed with 1 tbsp. lemon juice (100 calories)

347 calories

### Lunch

2 slices whole-grain bread spread with 2 tbsp. hummus and topped with 4 (¼ inch) round cucumber slices, ½ small sliced red bell pepper, and ¼ cup baby spinach (290 calories)

### Snack

1 orange with ½ cup blueberries (104 calories)

394 calories

### Dinner

Asparagus Cauliflower Pizza (page 238) (331 calories)

331 calories

### Treat

2 Strawberry Yogurt Ice Pops (page 267) (100 calories)

100 calories

**1,172 Total Calories**

## Day 26

### Breakfast

Berry Blaster Bowl (page 177) (273 calories)

### Snack

1 medium apple (95 calories)

368 calories

### Lunch

Strawberry Feta Summer Salad (page 211) with 1 slice whole-grain toast with butter (302 calories)

### Snack

4 tbsp. wasabi peas (90 calories)

392 calories

### Dinner

Pan-Seared Salmon Salad (page 231) with ¼ cup whole-grain brown rice (273 calories)

273 calories

### Treat

3 tbsp. whipped cream topped with ¼ cup blueberries and ½ cup sliced strawberries (81 calories)

81 calories

**1,114 Total Calories**

## Day 27

### Breakfast

2 slices vegan whole-wheat toast topped with 1 tbsp. peanut butter and ¼ cup sliced banana (247 calories)

### Snack

1 cup mixed berries tossed with 1 tbsp. lemon juice (100 calories)

347 calories

### Lunch

Sunshine Summer Salad (page 224) (289 calories)

### Snack

1 orange with ½ cup blueberries (104 calories)

393 calories

### Dinner

1 cup cooked whole-wheat pasta shells tossed with 1 cup arugula, 2 tbsp. shredded Romano cheese, ¼ cup cherry tomatoes, ½ tbsp. olive oil, and a dash of red pepper flakes (311 calories)

311 calories

### Treat

2 Strawberry Yogurt Ice Pops (page 267) (100 calories)

100 calories

**1,151 Total Calories**

## Day 28

### Breakfast

Berry Blaster Bowl (page 177) (273 calories)

### Snack

1 medium apple (95 calories)

368 calories

### Lunch

2 slices whole-grain bread spread with 2 tbsp. hummus and topped with 4 (¼ inch) round cucumber slices, ½ small sliced red bell pepper, and ¼ cup baby spinach (290 calories)

### Snack

4 tbsp. wasabi peas (90 calories)

380 calories

### Dinner

Asparagus Cauliflower Pizza (page 238) (331 calories)

331 calories

### Treat

3 tbsp. whipped cream topped with ¼ cup blueberries and ½ cup sliced strawberries (81 calories)

81 calories

**1,160 Total Calories**

## Day 29

### Breakfast

2 slices vegan whole-wheat toast topped with 1 tbsp. almond butter and ¼ cup halved strawberries (312 calories)

### Snack

¾ cup grapes (78 calories)

390 calories

### Lunch

Organic Chicken Caesar Salad (page 212) (310 calories)

### Snack

6 oz. plain Greek yogurt with 3 sliced strawberries (112 calories)

422 calories

### Dinner

3 oz. cooked wild salmon, ½ cup whole-grain brown rice, 1 cup sautéed kale, salt and pepper to taste (287 calories)

287 calories

### Treat

Banana Berry Ice Cream (page 255) (96 calories)

96 calories

**1,195 Total Calories**

## Day 30

### Breakfast

Tropical Mango Blast (page 169) (243 calories)

### Snack

1 orange with ½ cup blueberries (104 calories)

347 calories

### Lunch

Tomato Gazpacho Fresca (page 215) with 2 slices whole-wheat toast (346 calories)

### Snack

10 celery sticks with 1 tbsp. peanut butter (100 calories)

446 calories

### Dinner

Guilt-Free Zucchini Pasta (page 246) (222 calories)

222 calories

### Treat

6 oz. plain Greek yogurt mixed with cinnamon (100 calories)

100 calories

**1,115 Total Calories**

# Week 5

## Day 31

### Breakfast

2 slices vegan whole-wheat toast topped with 1 tbsp. almond butter and ¼ cup halved strawberries (312 calories)

### Snack

¾ cup grapes (78 calories)

390 calories

### Lunch

2 cups spinach tossed with 2 chopped hard-boiled eggs, ½ cup chopped red bell pepper, ½ cup sliced white mushrooms, ¼ cup avocado slices, and 2 tbsp. balsamic vinegar (283 calories)

### Snack

6 oz. plain Greek yogurt with 3 sliced strawberries (112 calories)

395 calories

### Dinner

California Fish Tacos (page 227) (251 calories)

251 calories

### Treat

Banana Berry Ice Cream (page 255) (96 calories)

96 calories

**1,132 Total Calories**

## Day 32

### Breakfast

Tropical Mango Blast (page 169) (243 calories)

### Snack

1 orange with ½ cup blueberries (104 calories)

347 calories

### Lunch

Organic Chicken Caesar Salad (page 212) (310 calories)

### Snack

10 celery sticks with 1 tbsp. peanut butter (100 calories)

410 calories

### Dinner

3 oz. cooked wild salmon, ½ cup whole-grain brown rice, 1 cup sautéed kale, salt and pepper to taste (287 calories)

287 calories

### Treat

6 oz. plain Greek yogurt mixed with cinnamon (100 calories)

100 calories

**1,144 Total Calories**

## Day 33

### Breakfast

2 slices vegan whole-wheat toast topped with 1 tbsp. almond butter and ¼ cup halved strawberries (312 calories)

### Snack

¾ cup grapes (78 calories)

390 calories

### Lunch

Tomato Gazpacho Fresca (page 215) with 2 slices whole-wheat toast (346 calories)

### Snack

6 oz. plain Greek yogurt with 3 sliced strawberries (112 calories)

458 calories

### Dinner

Guilt-Free Zucchini Pasta (page 246) (222 calories)

222 calories

### Treat

Banana Berry Ice Cream (page 255) (96 calories)

96 calories

**1,166 Total Calories**

## Day 34

### Breakfast

Tropical Mango Blast (page 169) (243 calories)

### Snack

1 orange with ½ cup blueberries (104 calories)

347 calories

### Lunch

2 cups spinach tossed with 2 chopped hard-boiled eggs, ½ cup chopped red bell pepper, ½ cup sliced white mushrooms, ¼ cup avocado slices, and 2 tbsp. balsamic vinegar (283 calories)

### Snack

10 celery sticks with 1 tbsp. peanut butter (100 calories)

383 calories

### Dinner

California Fish Tacos (page 227) (251 calories)

251 calories

### Treat

6 oz. plain Greek yogurt mixed with cinnamon (100 calories)

100 calories

**1,081 Total Calories**

## Week 5

### Day 35

#### Breakfast

2 slices vegan whole-wheat toast topped with 1 tbsp. almond butter and ¼ cup halved strawberries (312 calories)

#### Snack

¾ cup grapes (78 calories)

390 calories

#### Lunch

Organic Chicken Caesar Salad (page 212) (310 calories)

#### Snack

6 oz. plain Greek yogurt with 3 sliced strawberries (112 calories)

422 calories

#### Dinner

3 oz. cooked wild salmon, ½ cup whole-grain brown rice, 1 cup sautéed kale, salt and pepper to taste (287 calories)

287 calories

#### Treat

Banana Berry Ice Cream (page 255) (96 calories)

96 calories

**1,195 Total Calories**

## Week 6

### Day 36

#### Breakfast

Sunshine Cinnamon Nut Quinoa (page 189) (274 calories)

#### Snack

1 small banana (90 calories)

364 calories

#### Lunch

In a medium bowl, toss together ½ cup watermelon, ½ cup chopped cucumber, ¼ cup chopped avocado, and ¼ cup chopped radishes with 1 tsp. olive oil. Sprinkle with salt and pepper to taste. Serve with ½ cup Greek yogurt drizzled in 1 tsp. olive oil and salt and pepper. (243 calories)

#### Snack

15 baby carrots with 2 tbsp. tzatziki (83 calories)

326 calories

#### Dinner

Grilled Tilapia Grapefruit Salad (page 237) (260 calories)

260 calories

#### Treat

Cocoa Bean Brownie (page 256) (112 calories)

112 calories

**1,062 Total Calories**

# Week 6

## Day 37

### Breakfast

1 grapefruit with 1 slice vegan whole-wheat toast topped with 1 tbsp. almond butter (241 calories)

### Snack

1 medium apple (95 calories)

336 calories

### Lunch

Sweet Arugula Pear Salad (page 216) with 1 slice whole-grain toast (310 calories)

### Snack

1 cup blueberries (85 calories)

395 calories

### Dinner

3 oz. roasted chicken with 2 cups roasted vegetables and ½ baked sweet potato (272 calories)

272 calories

### Treat

2 tbsp. light whipped cream topped with 1 cup sliced strawberries and ¼ sliced banana (90 calories)

90 calories

**1,093 Total Calories**

## Day 38

### Breakfast

Sunshine Cinnamon Nut Quinoa (page 189) (274 calories)

### Snack

1 small banana (90 calories)

364 calories

### Lunch

Garden Greek Salad (page 245) (312 calories)

### Snack

15 baby carrots with 2 tbsp. tzatziki (83 calories)

395 calories

### Dinner

Spaghetti Squash Pasta (page 250) (300 calories)

300 calories

### Treat

Cocoa Bean Brownie (page 256) (112 calories)

112 calories

**1,171 Total Calories**

## Day 39

### Breakfast

1 grapefruit with 1 slice vegan whole-wheat toast topped with 1 tbsp. almond butter (241 calories)

### Snack

1 medium apple (95 calories)

336 calories

### Lunch

In a medium bowl, toss together ½ cup watermelon, ½ cup chopped cucumber, ¼ cup chopped avocado, and ¼ cup chopped radishes with 1 tsp. olive oil. Sprinkle with salt and pepper to taste. Serve with ½ cup Greek yogurt drizzled in 1 tsp. olive oil and salt and pepper. (243 calories)

### Snack

1 cup blueberries (85 calories)

328 calories

### Dinner

Grilled Tilapia Grapefruit Salad (page 237) (260 calories)

260 calories

### Treat

2 tbsp. light whipped cream topped with 1 cup sliced strawberries and ¼ sliced banana (90 calories)

90 calories

**1,014 Total Calories**

## Day 40

### Breakfast

Sunshine Cinnamon Nut Quinoa (page 189) (274 calories)

### Snack

1 small banana (90 calories)

364 calories

### Lunch

Sweet Arugula Pear Salad (page 216) with 1 slice whole-grain toast (310 calories)

### Snack

15 baby carrots with 2 tbsp. tzatziki (83 calories)

393 calories

### Dinner

3 oz. roasted chicken with 2 cups roasted vegetables and ½ baked sweet potato (272 calories)

272 calories

### Treat

Cocoa Bean Brownie (page 256) (112 calories)

112 calories

**1,141 Total Calories**

## Day 41

### Breakfast

1 grapefruit with 1 slice vegan whole-wheat toast topped with 1 tbsp. almond butter (241 calories)

### Snack

1 medium apple (95 calories)

336 calories

### Lunch

Garden Greek Salad (page 245) (312 calories)

### Snack

1 cup blueberries (85 calories)

397 calories

### Dinner

Spaghetti Squash Pasta (page 250) (300 calories)

300 calories

### Treat

2 tbsp. light whipped cream topped with 1 cup sliced strawberries and ¼ sliced banana (90 calories)

90 calories

**1,123 Total Calories**

## Day 42

### Breakfast

Sunshine Cinnamon Nut Quinoa (page 189) (274 calories)

### Snack

1 small banana (90 calories)

364 calories

### Lunch

In a medium bowl, toss together ½ cup watermelon, ½ cup chopped cucumber, ¼ cup chopped avocado, and ¼ cup chopped radishes with 1 tsp. olive oil. Sprinkle with salt and pepper to taste. Serve with ½ cup Greek yogurt drizzled in 1 tsp. olive oil and salt and pepper. (243 calories)

### Snack

15 baby carrots with 2 tbsp. tzatziki (83 calories)

326 calories

### Dinner

Grilled Tilapia Grapefruit Salad (page 237) (260 calories)

260 calories

### Treat

Cocoa Bean Brownie (page 256) (112 calories)

112 calories

**1,062 Total Calories**

## Day 43

### Breakfast

½ cup rolled oats with ½ cup raspberries and 1 cup unsweetened almond milk (252 calories)

### Snack

1 cup unsweetened applesauce sprinkled with cinnamon (100 calories)

352 calories

### Lunch

Turkocado Salad (page 219) (238 calories)

### Snack

1 cup cherries (95 calories)

352 calories

### Dinner

Baked Cauliflower Casserole (page 241) (250 calories)

250 calories

### Treat

2 slices Watermelon Lover's Pizza (page 272) with 3 oz. plain Greek yogurt (102 calories)

102 calories

**1,037 Total Calories**

## Day 44

### Breakfast

Sweet Greens Smoothie Bowl (page 181) (341 calories)

### Snack

4 medium strawberries dipped in 1 tbsp. melted dark chocolate (100 calories)

441 calories

### Lunch

1 small whole-wheat roll filled with 2 oz. grilled chicken, 1 leaf romaine lettuce, 1 slice tomato, and 1 tsp. mustard (276 calories)

### Snack

6 oz. plain Greek yogurt topped with 3 raspberries (103 calories)

379 calories

### Dinner

Sunshine Summer Salad (page 224) (289 calories)

289 calories

### Treat

1 medium frozen banana pureed into ice cream (105 calories)

105 calories

**1,214 Total Calories**

## Day 45

### Breakfast

½ cup rolled oats with ½ cup raspberries and 1 cup unsweetened almond milk (252 calories)

### Snack

1 cup unsweetened applesauce sprinkled with cinnamon (100 calories)

352 calories

### Lunch

Organic Artichoke Tomato Soup (page 249) (200 calories)

### Snack

1 cup cherries (95 calories)

295 calories

### Dinner

3 oz. roasted turkey breast, ½ cup sautéed mushrooms, ½ cup whole-grain brown rice, 1 pat butter (286 calories)

286 calories

### Treat

2 slices Watermelon Lover's Pizza (page 272) with 3 oz. plain Greek yogurt (102 calories)

102 calories

**1,035 Total Calories**

## Day 46

### Breakfast

Sweet Greens Smoothie Bowl (page 181) (341 calories)

### Snack

4 medium strawberries dipped in 1 tbsp. melted dark chocolate (100 calories)

441 calories

### Lunch

Turkocado Salad (page 219) (238 calories)

### Snack

6 oz. plain Greek yogurt topped with 3 raspberries (103 calories)

341 calories

### Dinner

Baked Cauliflower Casserole (page 241) (250 calories)

250 calories

### Treat

1 medium frozen banana pureed into ice cream (105 calories)

105 calories

**1,137 Total Calories**

## Day 47

### Breakfast

½ cup rolled oats with ½ cup raspberries and 1 cup unsweetened almond milk (252 calories)

### Snack

1 cup unsweetened applesauce sprinkled with cinnamon (100 calories)

352 calories

### Lunch

1 small whole-wheat roll filled with 2 oz. grilled chicken, 1 leaf romaine lettuce, 1 slice tomato, and 1 tsp. mustard (276 calories)

### Snack

1 cup cherries (95 calories)

371 calories

### Dinner

Sunshine Summer Salad (page 224) (289 calories)

289 calories

### Treat

2 slices Watermelon Lover's Pizza (page 272) with 3 oz. plain Greek yogurt (102 calories)

102 calories

**1,114 Total Calories**

## Day 48

### Breakfast

Sweet Greens Smoothie Bowl (page 181) (341 calories)

### Snack

4 medium strawberries dipped in 1 tbsp. melted dark chocolate (100 calories)

441 calories

### Lunch

Organic Artichoke Tomato Soup (page 249) (200 calories)

### Snack

6 oz. plain Greek yogurt topped with 3 raspberries (103 calories)

303 calories

### Dinner

3 oz. roasted turkey breast, ½ cup sautéed mushrooms, ½ cup whole-grain brown rice, 1 pat butter (286 calories)

286 calories

### Treat

1 medium frozen banana pureed into ice cream (105 calories)

105 calories

**1,135 Total Calories**

## Day 49

### Breakfast

½ cup rolled oats with ½ cup raspberries and 1 cup unsweetened almond milk (252 calories)

### Snack

1 cup unsweetened applesauce sprinkled with cinnamon (100 calories)

352 calories

### Lunch

Turkocado Salad (page 219) (238 calories)

### Snack

1 cup cherries (95 calories)

333 calories

### Dinner

Baked Cauliflower Casserole (page 241) (250 calories)

250 calories

### Treat

2 slices Watermelon Lover's Pizza (page 272) with 3 oz. plain Greek yogurt (102 calories)

102 calories

**1,037 Total Calories**

## Day 50

### Breakfast

Berry Blaster Bowl (page 177) (273 calories)

### Snack

1 medium apple (95 calories)

368 calories

### Lunch

2 slices whole-grain bread spread with 2 tbsp. hummus and topped with 4 (¼ inch) round cucumber slices, ½ small sliced red bell pepper, and ¼ cup baby spinach (290 calories)

### Snack

4 tbsp. wasabi peas (90 calories)

380 calories

### Dinner

Asparagus Cauliflower Pizza (page 238) (331 calories)

331 calories

### Treat

3 tbsp. whipped cream topped with ¼ cup blueberries and ½ cup sliced strawberries (81 calories)

81 calories

**1,160 Total Calories**

## Day 51

### Breakfast

2 slices vegan whole-wheat toast topped with 1 tbsp. peanut butter and ¼ cup sliced banana (247 calories)

### Snack

1 cup mixed berries tossed with 1 tbsp. lemon juice (100 calories)

347 calories

### Lunch

Strawberry Feta Summer Salad (page 211) with 1 slice whole-grain toast with butter (302 calories)

### Snack

1 orange with ½ cup blueberries (104 calories)

406 calories

### Dinner

Pan-Seared Salmon Salad (page 231) with ¼ cup whole-grain brown rice (273 calories)

273 calories

### Treat

2 Strawberry Yogurt Ice Pops (page 267) (100 calories)

100 calories

**1,126 Total Calories**

## Day 52

### Breakfast

Berry Blaster Bowl (page 177) (273 calories)

### Snack

1 medium apple (95 calories)

368 calories

### Lunch

Sunshine Summer Salad (page 224) (289 calories)

### Snack

4 tbsp. wasabi peas (90 calories)

379 calories

### Dinner

1 cup cooked whole-wheat pasta shells tossed with 1 cup arugula, 2 tbsp. shredded Romano cheese, ¼ cup cherry tomatoes, ½ tbsp. olive oil, and a dash of red pepper flakes (311 calories)

311 calories

### Treat

3 tbsp. whipped cream topped with ¼ cup blueberries and ½ cup sliced strawberries (81 calories)

81 calories

**1,139 Total Calories**

## Day 53

### Breakfast

2 slices vegan whole-wheat toast topped with 1 tbsp. peanut butter and ¼ cup sliced banana (247 calories)

### Snack

1 cup mixed berries tossed with 1 tbsp. lemon juice (100 calories)

347 calories

### Lunch

2 slices whole-grain bread spread with 2 tbsp. hummus and topped with 4 (¼ inch) round cucumber slices, ½ small sliced red bell pepper, and ¼ cup baby spinach (290 calories)

### Snack

1 orange with ½ cup blueberries (104 calories)

394 calories

### Dinner

Asparagus Cauliflower Pizza (page 238) (331 calories)

331 calories

### Treat

2 Strawberry Yogurt Ice Pops (page 267) (100 calories)

100 calories

**1,172 Total Calories**

## Day 54

### Breakfast

Berry Blaster Bowl (page 177) (273 calories)

### Snack

1 medium apple (95 calories)

368 calories

### Lunch

Strawberry Feta Summer Salad (page 211) with 1 slice whole-grain toast with butter (302 calories)

### Snack

4 tbsp. wasabi peas (90 calories)

392 calories

### Dinner

Pan-Seared Salmon Salad (page 231) with ¼ cup whole-grain brown rice (273 calories)

273 calories

### Treat

3 tbsp. whipped cream topped with ¼ cup blueberries and ½ cup sliced strawberries (81 calories)

81 calories

**1,114 Total Calories**

## Day 55

### Breakfast

2 slices vegan whole-wheat toast topped with 1 tbsp. peanut butter and ¼ cup sliced banana (247 calories)

### Snack

1 cup mixed berries tossed with 1 tbsp. lemon juice (100 calories)

347 calories

### Lunch

Sunshine Summer Salad (page 224) (289 calories)

### Snack

1 orange with ½ cup blueberries (104 calories)

393 calories

### Dinner

1 cup cooked whole-wheat pasta shells tossed with 1 cup arugula, 2 tbsp. shredded Romano cheese, ¼ cup cherry tomatoes, ½ tbsp. olive oil, and a dash of red pepper flakes (311 calories)

311 calories

### Treat

2 Strawberry Yogurt Ice Pops (page 267) (100 calories)

100 calories

**1,151 Total Calories**

## Day 56

### Breakfast

Berry Blaster Bowl (page 177) (273 calories)

### Snack

1 medium apple (95 calories)

368 calories

### Lunch

2 slices whole-grain bread spread with 2 tbsp. hummus and topped with 4 (¼ inch) round cucumber slices, ½ small sliced red bell pepper, and ¼ cup baby spinach (290 calories)

### Snack

4 tbsp. wasabi peas (90 calories)

380 calories

### Dinner

Asparagus Cauliflower Pizza (page 238) (331 calories)

331 calories

### Treat

3 tbsp. whipped cream topped with ¼ cup blueberries and ½ cup sliced strawberries (81 calories)

81 calories

**1,160 Total Calories**

## Day 57

### Breakfast

2 slices vegan whole-wheat toast topped with 1 tbsp. almond butter and ¼ cup halved strawberries (312 calories)

### Snack

¾ cup grapes (78 calories)

390 calories

### Lunch

Organic Chicken Caesar Salad (page 212) (310 calories)

### Snack

6 oz. plain Greek yogurt with 3 sliced strawberries (112 calories)

422 calories

### Dinner

3 oz. cooked wild salmon, ½ cup whole-grain brown rice, 1 cup sautéed kale, salt and pepper to taste (287 calories)

287 calories

### Treat

Banana Berry Ice Cream (page 255) (96 calories)

96 calories

**1,195 Total Calories**

## Day 58

### Breakfast

Tropical Mango Blast (page 169) (243 calories)

### Snack

1 orange with ½ cup blueberries (104 calories)

347 calories

### Lunch

Tomato Gazpacho Fresca (page 215) with 2 slices whole-wheat toast (346 calories)

### Snack

10 celery sticks with 1 tbsp. peanut butter (100 calories)

446 calories

### Dinner

Guilt-Free Zucchini Pasta (page 246) (222 calories)

222 calories

### Treat

6 oz. plain Greek yogurt mixed with cinnamon (100 calories)

100 calories

**1,115 Total Calories**

## Day 59

### Breakfast

2 slices vegan whole-wheat toast topped with 1 tbsp. almond butter and ¼ cup halved strawberries (312 calories)

### Snack

¾ cup grapes (78 calories)

390 calories

### Lunch

2 cups spinach tossed with 2 chopped hard-boiled eggs, ½ cup chopped red bell pepper, ½ cup sliced white mushrooms, ¼ cup avocado slices, and 2 tbsp. balsamic vinegar (283 calories)

### Snack

6 oz. plain Greek yogurt with 3 sliced strawberries (112 calories)

395 calories

### Dinner

California Fish Tacos (page 227) (251 calories)

251 calories

### Treat

Banana Berry Ice Cream (page 255) (96 calories)

96 calories

**1,132 Total Calories**

## Day 60

### Breakfast

Tropical Mango Blast (page 169) (243 calories)

### Snack

1 orange with ½ cup blueberries (104 calories)

347 calories

### Lunch

Organic Chicken Caesar Salad (page 212) (310 calories)

### Snack

10 celery sticks with 1 tbsp. peanut butter (100 calories)

410 calories

### Dinner

3 oz. cooked wild salmon, ½ cup whole-grain brown rice, 1 cup sautéed kale, salt and pepper to taste (287 calories)

287 calories

### Treat

6 oz. plain Greek yogurt mixed with cinnamon (100 calories)

100 calories

**1,144 Total Calories**

# Week 9

## Day 61

### Breakfast

2 slices vegan whole-wheat toast topped with 1 tbsp. almond butter and ¼ cup halved strawberries (312 calories)

### Snack

¾ cup grapes (78 calories)

390 calories

### Lunch

Tomato Gazpacho Fresca (page 215) with 2 slices whole-wheat toast (346 calories)

### Snack

6 oz. plain Greek yogurt with 3 sliced strawberries (112 calories)

458 calories

### Dinner

Guilt-Free Zucchini Pasta (page 246) (222 calories)

222 calories

### Treat

Banana Berry Ice Cream (page 255) (96 calories)

96 calories

**1,166 Total Calories**

## Day 62

### Breakfast

Tropical Mango Blast (page 169) (243 calories)

### Snack

1 orange with ½ cup blueberries (104 calories)

347 calories

### Lunch

2 cups spinach tossed with 2 chopped hard-boiled eggs, ½ cup chopped red bell pepper, ½ cup sliced white mushrooms, ¼ cup avocado slices, and 2 tbsp. balsamic vinegar (283 calories)

### Snack

10 celery sticks with 1 tbsp. peanut butter (100 calories)

383 calories

### Dinner

California Fish Tacos (page 227) (251 calories)

251 calories

### Treat

6 oz. plain Greek yogurt mixed with cinnamon (100 calories)

100 calories

**1,081 Total Calories**

### Day 63

**Breakfast**

2 slices vegan whole-wheat toast topped with 1 tbsp. almond butter and ¼ cup halved strawberries (312 calories)

**Snack**

¾ cup grapes (78 calories)

390 calories

**Lunch**

Organic Chicken Caesar Salad (page 212) (310 calories)

**Snack**

6 oz. plain Greek yogurt with 3 sliced strawberries (112 calories)

422 calories

**Dinner**

3 oz. cooked wild salmon, ½ cup whole-grain brown rice, 1 cup sautéed kale, salt and pepper to taste (287 calories)

287 calories

**Treat**

Banana Berry Ice Cream (page 255) (96 calories)

96 calories

**1,195 Total Calories**

### Day 64

**Breakfast**

Sunshine Cinnamon Nut Quinoa (page 189) (274 calories)

**Snack**

1 small banana (90 calories)

364 calories

**Lunch**

In a medium bowl, toss together ½ cup watermelon, ½ cup chopped cucumber, ¼ cup chopped avocado, and ¼ cup chopped radishes with 1 tsp. olive oil. Sprinkle with salt and pepper to taste. Serve with ½ cup Greek yogurt drizzled in 1 tsp. olive oil and salt and pepper. (243 calories)

**Snack**

15 baby carrots with 2 tbsp. tzatziki (83 calories)

326 calories

**Dinner**

Grilled Tilapia Grapefruit Salad (page 237) (260 calories)

260 calories

**Treat**

Cocoa Bean Brownie (page 256) (112 calories)

112 calories

**1,062 Total Calories**

## Day 65

### Breakfast

1 grapefruit with 1 slice vegan whole-wheat toast topped with 1 tbsp. almond butter (241 calories)

### Snack

1 medium apple (95 calories)

336 calories

### Lunch

Sweet Arugula Pear Salad (page 216) with 1 slice whole-grain toast (310 calories)

### Snack

1 cup blueberries (85 calories)

395 calories

### Dinner

3 oz. roasted chicken with 2 cups roasted vegetables and ½ baked sweet potato (272 calories)

272 calories

### Treat

2 tbsp. light whipped cream topped with 1 cup sliced strawberries and ¼ sliced banana (90 calories)

90 calories

**1,093 Total Calories**

## Day 66

### Breakfast

Sunshine Cinnamon Nut Quinoa (page 189) (274 calories)

### Snack

1 small banana (90 calories)

364 calories

### Lunch

Garden Greek Salad (page 245) (312 calories)

### Snack

15 baby carrots with 2 tbsp. tzatziki (83 calories)

395 calories

### Dinner

Spaghetti Squash Pasta (page 250) (300 calories)

300 calories

### Treat

Cocoa Bean Brownie (page 256) (112 calories)

112 calories

**1,171 Total Calories**

## Day 67

### Breakfast

1 grapefruit with 1 slice vegan whole-wheat toast topped with 1 tbsp. almond butter (241 calories)

### Snack

1 medium apple (95 calories)

336 calories

### Lunch

In a medium bowl, toss together ½ cup watermelon, ½ cup chopped cucumber, ¼ cup chopped avocado, and ¼ cup chopped radishes with 1 tsp. olive oil. Sprinkle with salt and pepper to taste. Serve with ½ cup Greek yogurt drizzled in 1 tsp. olive oil and salt and pepper. (243 calories)

### Snack

1 cup blueberries (85 calories)

328 calories

### Dinner

Grilled Tilapia Grapefruit Salad (page 237) (260 calories)

260 calories

### Treat

2 tbsp. light whipped cream topped with 1 cup sliced strawberries and ¼ sliced banana (90 calories)

90 calories

**1,014 Total Calories**

## Day 68

### Breakfast

Sunshine Cinnamon Nut Quinoa (page 189) (274 calories)

### Snack

1 small banana (90 calories)

364 calories

### Lunch

Sweet Arugula Pear Salad (page 216) with 1 slice whole-grain toast (310 calories)

### Snack

15 baby carrots with 2 tbsp. tzatziki (83 calories)

393 calories

### Dinner

3 oz. roasted chicken with 2 cups roasted vegetables and ½ baked sweet potato (272 calories)

272 calories

### Treat

Cocoa Bean Brownie (page 256) (112 calories)

112 calories

**1,141 Total Calories**

## Day 69

### Breakfast

1 grapefruit with 1 slice vegan whole-wheat toast topped with 1 tbsp. almond butter (241 calories)

### Snack

1 medium apple (95 calories)

336 calories

### Lunch

Garden Greek Salad (page 245) (312 calories)

### Snack

1 cup blueberries (85 calories)

397 calories

### Dinner

Spaghetti Squash Pasta (page 250) (300 calories)

300 calories

### Treat

2 tbsp. light whipped cream topped with 1 cup sliced strawberries and ¼ sliced banana (90 calories)

90 calories

**1,123 Total Calories**

## Day 70

### Breakfast

Sunshine Cinnamon Nut Quinoa (page 189) (274 calories)

### Snack

1 small banana (90 calories)

364 calories

### Lunch

In a medium bowl, toss together ½ cup watermelon, ½ cup chopped cucumber, ¼ cup chopped avocado, and ¼ cup chopped radishes with 1 tsp. olive oil. Sprinkle with salt and pepper to taste. Serve with ½ cup Greek yogurt drizzled in 1 tsp. olive oil and salt and pepper. (243 calories)

### Snack

15 baby carrots with 2 tbsp. tzatziki (83 calories)

326 calories

### Dinner

Grilled Tilapia Grapefruit Salad (page 237) (260 calories)

260 calories

### Treat

Cocoa Bean Brownie (page 256) (112 calories)

112 calories

**1,062 Total Calories**

## Day 71

### Breakfast

½ cup rolled oats with ½ cup raspberries and 1 cup unsweetened almond milk (252 calories)

### Snack

1 cup unsweetened applesauce sprinkled with cinnamon (100 calories)

352 calories

### Lunch

Turkocado Salad (page 219) (238 calories)

### Snack

1 cup cherries (95 calories)

333 calories

### Dinner

Baked Cauliflower Casserole (page 241) (250 calories)

250 calories

### Treat

2 slices Watermelon Lover's Pizza (page 272) with 3 oz. plain Greek yogurt (102 calories)

102 calories

**1,037 Total Calories**

## Day 72

### Breakfast

Sweet Greens Smoothie Bowl (page 181) (341 calories)

### Snack

4 medium strawberries dipped in 1 tbsp. melted dark chocolate (100 calories)

441 calories

### Lunch

1 small whole-wheat roll filled with 2 oz. grilled chicken, 1 leaf romaine lettuce, 1 slice tomato, and 1 tsp. mustard (276 calories)

### Snack

6 oz. plain Greek yogurt topped with 3 raspberries (103 calories)

379 calories

### Dinner

Sunshine Summer Salad (page 224) (289 calories)

289 calories

### Treat

1 medium frozen banana pureed into ice cream (105 calories)

105 calories

**1,214 Total Calories**

## Day 73

### Breakfast

½ cup rolled oats with ½ cup raspberries and 1 cup unsweetened almond milk (252 calories)

### Snack

1 cup unsweetened applesauce sprinkled with cinnamon (100 calories)

352 calories

### Lunch

Organic Artichoke Tomato Soup (page 249) (200 calories)

### Snack

1 cup cherries (95 calories)

295 calories

### Dinner

3 oz. roasted turkey breast, ½ cup sautéed mushrooms, ½ cup whole-grain brown rice, 1 pat butter (286 calories)

286 calories

### Treat

2 slices Watermelon Lover's Pizza (page 272) with 3 oz. plain Greek yogurt (102 calories)

102 calories

**1,035 Total Calories**

## Day 74

### Breakfast

Sweet Greens Smoothie Bowl (page 181) (341 calories)

### Snack

4 medium strawberries dipped in 1 tbsp. melted dark chocolate (100 calories)

441 calories

### Lunch

Turkocado Salad (page 219) (238 calories)

### Snack

6 oz. plain Greek yogurt topped with 3 raspberries (103 calories)

341 calories

### Dinner

Baked Cauliflower Casserole (page 241) (250 calories)

250 calories

### Treat

1 medium frozen banana pureed into ice cream (105 calories)

105 calories

**1,137 Total Calories**

## Day 75

### Breakfast

½ cup rolled oats with ½ cup raspberries and 1 cup unsweetened almond milk (252 calories)

### Snack

1 cup unsweetened applesauce sprinkled with cinnamon (100 calories)

352 calories

### Lunch

1 small whole-wheat roll filled with 2 oz. grilled chicken, 1 leaf romaine lettuce, 1 slice tomato, and 1 tsp. mustard (276 calories)

### Snack

1 cup cherries (95 calories)

371 calories

### Dinner

Sunshine Summer Salad (page 224) (289 calories)

289 calories

### Treat

2 slices Watermelon Lover's Pizza (page 272) with 3 oz. plain Greek yogurt (102 calories)

102 calories

**1,114 Total Calories**

## Day 76

### Breakfast

Sweet Greens Smoothie Bowl (page 181) (341 calories)

### Snack

4 medium strawberries dipped in 1 tbsp. melted dark chocolate (100 calories)

441 calories

### Lunch

Organic Artichoke Tomato Soup (page 249) (200 calories)

### Snack

6 oz. plain Greek yogurt topped with 3 raspberries (103 calories)

303 calories

### Dinner

3 oz. roasted turkey breast, ½ cup sautéed mushrooms, ½ cup whole-grain brown rice, 1 pat butter (286 calories)

286 calories

### Treat

1 medium frozen banana pureed into ice cream (105 calories)

105 calories

**1,135 Total Calories**

## Week 11

### Day 77

#### Breakfast

½ cup rolled oats with ½ cup raspberries and 1 cup unsweetened almond milk (252 calories)

#### Snack

1 cup unsweetened applesauce sprinkled with cinnamon (100 calories)

352 calories

#### Lunch

Turkocado Salad (page 219) (238 calories)

#### Snack

1 cup cherries (95 calories)

333 calories

#### Dinner

Baked Cauliflower Casserole (page 241) (250 calories)

250 calories

#### Treat

2 slices Watermelon Lover's Pizza (page 272) with 3 oz. plain Greek yogurt (102 calories)

102 calories

**1,037 Total Calories**

## Week 12

### Day 78

#### Breakfast

Berry Blaster Bowl (page 177) (273 calories)

#### Snack

1 medium apple (95 calories)

368 calories

#### Lunch

2 slices whole-grain bread spread with 2 tbsp. hummus and topped with 4 (¼ inch) round cucumber slices, ½ small sliced red bell pepper, and ¼ cup baby spinach (290 calories)

#### Snack

4 tbsp. wasabi peas (90 calories)

380 calories

#### Dinner

Asparagus Cauliflower Pizza (page 238) (331 calories)

331 calories

#### Treat

3 tbsp. whipped cream topped with ¼ cup blueberries and ½ cup sliced strawberries (81 calories)

81 calories

**1,160 Total Calories**

## Day 79

### Breakfast

2 slices vegan whole-wheat toast topped with 1 tbsp. peanut butter and ¼ cup sliced banana (247 calories)

### Snack

1 cup mixed berries tossed with 1 tbsp. lemon juice (100 calories)

347 calories

### Lunch

Strawberry Feta Summer Salad (page 211) with 1 slice whole-grain toast with butter (302 calories)

### Snack

1 orange with ½ cup blueberries (104 calories)

406 calories

### Dinner

Pan-Seared Salmon Salad (page 231) with ¼ cup whole-grain brown rice (273 calories)

273 calories

### Treat

2 Strawberry Yogurt Ice Pops (page 267) (100 calories)

100 calories

**1,126 Total Calories**

## Day 80

### Breakfast

Berry Blaster Bowl (page 177) (273 calories)

### Snack

1 medium apple (95 calories)

368 calories

### Lunch

Sunshine Summer Salad (page 224) (289 calories)

### Snack

4 tbsp. wasabi peas (90 calories)

379 calories

### Dinner

1 cup cooked whole-wheat pasta shells tossed with 1 cup arugula, 2 tbsp. shredded Romano cheese, ¼ cup cherry tomatoes, ½ tbsp. olive oil, and a dash of red pepper flakes (311 calories)

311 calories

### Treat

3 tbsp. whipped cream topped with ¼ cup blueberries and ½ cup sliced strawberries (81 calories)

81 calories

**1,139 Total Calories**

## Day 81

### Breakfast

2 slices vegan whole-wheat toast topped with 1 tbsp. peanut butter and ¼ cup sliced banana (247 calories)

### Snack

1 cup mixed berries tossed with 1 tbsp. lemon juice (100 calories)

347 calories

### Lunch

2 slices whole-grain bread spread with 2 tbsp. hummus and topped with 4 (¼ inch) round cucumber slices, ½ small sliced red bell pepper, and ¼ cup baby spinach (290 calories)

### Snack

1 orange with ½ cup blueberries (104 calories)

394 calories

### Dinner

Asparagus Cauliflower Pizza (page 238) (331 calories)

331 calories

### Treat

2 Strawberry Yogurt Ice Pops (page 267) (100 calories)

100 calories

**1,172 Total Calories**

## Day 82

### Breakfast

Berry Blaster Bowl (page 177) (273 calories)

### Snack

1 medium apple (95 calories)

368 calories

### Lunch

Strawberry Feta Summer Salad (page 211) with 1 slice whole-grain toast with butter (302 calories)

### Snack

4 tbsp. wasabi peas (90 calories)

392 calories

### Dinner

Pan-Seared Salmon Salad (page 231) with ¼ cup whole-grain brown rice (273 calories)

273 calories

### Treat

3 tbsp. whipped cream topped with ¼ cup blueberries and ½ cup sliced strawberries (81 calories)

81 calories

**1,114 Total Calories**

## Day 83

### Breakfast

2 slices vegan whole-wheat toast topped with 1 tbsp. peanut butter and ¼ cup sliced banana (247 calories)

### Snack

1 cup mixed berries tossed with 1 tbsp. lemon juice (100 calories)

347 calories

### Lunch

Sunshine Summer Salad (page 224) (289 calories)

### Snack

1 orange with ½ cup blueberries (104 calories)

393 calories

### Dinner

1 cup cooked whole-wheat pasta shells tossed with 1 cup arugula, 2 tbsp. shredded Romano cheese, ¼ cup cherry tomatoes, ½ tbsp. olive oil, and a dash of red pepper flakes (311 calories)

311 calories

### Treat

2 Strawberry Yogurt Ice Pops (page 267) (100 calories)

100 calories

**1,151 Total Calories**

## Day 84

### Breakfast

Berry Blaster Bowl (page 177) (273 calories)

### Snack

1 medium apple (95 calories)

368 calories

### Lunch

2 slices whole-grain bread spread with 2 tbsp. hummus and topped with 4 (¼ inch) round cucumber slices, ½ small sliced red bell pepper, and ¼ cup baby spinach (290 calories)

### Snack

4 tbsp. wasabi peas (90 calories)

380 calories

### Dinner

Asparagus Cauliflower Pizza (page 238) (331 calories)

331 calories

### Treat

3 tbsp. whipped cream topped with ¼ cup blueberries and ½ cup sliced strawberries (81 calories)

81 calories

**1,160 Total Calories**

# 5 Your 12-Week Fitness Guide

A s a celebrity fitness trainer, I know the stigmas that come with working out. People often picture gym memberships and personal trainers, spending mindless hours on the elliptical, crunches upon crunches . . . the list could go on. While there are those who enjoy this type of exercise, it's not for everyone. It's also not required for true health and fitness.

My philosophy as a fitness trainer has always been to keep it simple. I believe that a healthier, more fit you all comes down to *three things,* and three things only. Sit less, move more, and exercise.

Let's start with the simplest one: *sit less.* Sounds easy enough, right? Well it is. All it requires is standing up more throughout the day. The average person sits for 7.7 hours or more each day—commuting to work, sitting at your desk, sitting at home. That's a lot of sitting! Those of you with desk jobs know this all too well. However, all you need to do is commit to standing up once every hour. Go down the hall and grab a cup of coffee, take a restroom break, do a lap around the cubicles and say hi to your coworkers. You can even just stand up at your desk for a few minutes to stretch your legs. That's all it takes. This simple movement will help keep your lower body more toned and keep your metabolism going. All too many of my clients suffer from a broken metabolism because they simply do not stand up enough.

The next step is to *move more.* This comes down to knowing how many steps you take each day. I highly recommend getting a pedometer or using an app or fitness tracker. Not enough people use pedometers these days but they are incredibly helpful in making sure your body is staying active. The common goal to shoot for is 10,000 steps per day. For a fairly active person, this is no big deal. However, if you start tracking your steps and realize you are way under, aim to increase your daily steps by 1,000 until you reach 10,000. Some simple ways to up your step count include parking the car further away from the grocery store entrance, taking the dog twice around the block instead of once, or walking to your lunch spot down the street from the office instead of driving. Start small and work your way up.

The third and final step is to *get some exercise.* This one can be a little tougher, especially because it takes time. We are all so busy, finding time for a workout often comes last. However, it is vital to carve out at least 20 minutes of cardiovascular exercise a day. This can be walking, jogging, rowing, cycling, etc. Anything that gets your heart rate up. I enjoy doing cardio as well as strength training in the form of High Intensity Interval Training (HIIT). I believe this type of exercise is extremely beneficial because it's not only cardiovascular exercise, but it helps tone your muscles as well.

That is why I am thrilled to introduce to you my Tiny and Full Workouts! Beyond just helping you get in your exercise, the workouts I'm about to show you come from absolute, unequivocal evidence that you can—and will—trigger your body's most aggressive belly fat-burning mechanisms.

Here's a brief chemistry lesson: To burn off fat, your body creates an enzyme called hormone-sensitive lipase (HSL). HSL breaks down fat and tells your body to burn it up as fuel. If your body isn't making a whole lot of HSL, you're not going to break down much fat. If HSL levels are high, your body becomes a fat-burning furnace. A

## Why Most Exercise Fails at Burning Fat

Many health experts recommend that you get an hour or more of moderate-level exercise each day. But did you know that hour is really intended to maintain weight and health, not to lose fat or inches and not to fight disease? There is actually no research that backs up using this type of exercise specifically for weight loss. I'm not saying that exercising for an hour a day is bad for you—it's certainly not. Any time you move, your mental and physical health will benefit. But your belly fat will still be there.

whole bunch of hormones have an effect on HSL—testosterone, cortisol, estrogen, and human growth hormone—but the most distinctive are catecholamines.

Catecholamines are a group of hormones, including dopamine, histamine, adrenaline, and more, that unleash HSL like nothing else. The most important of these for our fat-burning purposes is adrenaline, which is the main hormone released when we are triggered by a threat, surprise, or danger—often referred to as the fight or flight response. During this reaction, adrenaline is released, speeding the heart rate, slowing digestion, shunting blood flow to major muscle groups, and changing various other nervous system functions. When this happens, it gives your body a burst of energy and strength. It's this reaction that pushes your body into a state where fat stores start breaking down so that they can be used for fuel.

Here's the scenario: Your body believes it's in danger, it's stressed, and it knows that it has to do everything possible to protect and save itself. So what does it do? Your body releases all the fat possible so it can start using it as fuel and keep you going even if you don't have the energy to do it for yourself.

That very same adrenaline makes it possible to spot-reduce your abdominal area because your belly region is loaded with more catecholamine receptors than any other part of your body. In other words, you have your own personal army of fat burners living right there in the place they're needed the most. But if you're used to doing cardio on cruise control—or not exercising at all—your army has been doing a lot more snoozing than fighting. So how do we wake it up without actually putting you in grave danger? Catecholamines respond most to one type of exercise technique, which is the very basis for the exercise routines here. This type of exercise is called High-Intensity Interval Training (HIIT). According to a groundbreaking study published in the *Journal of Obesity*, at the University of South Wales, women who performed HIIT just three times a week lost more subcutaneous and abdominal fat than those who did low-impact exercise. They spot-reduced their belly fat, which isn't supposed to be possible according to older research, but now we know that HIIT stimulates the catecholamine receptors in your abdominal muscles. You turn on the receptors and the adrenaline mobilizes the fat in your belly and burns it up during your workout.

HIIT is more often referred to as intense interval training, which is simply a workout made up of alternating short intense anaerobic exercise with less intense recovery periods. I've designed these workouts to do just this. You'll simply perform the four circuit exercises for 7 minutes, take a quick rest, then perform the other four circuit exercises for another 7 minutes, rest, and repeat the entire workout a second time. By doing this just three times a week, you'll burn belly fat, boost your heart rate, and condition every muscle in your body. This is all it takes to set off catecholamines, especially adrenaline, and start burning belly fat.

Do these moves three times a week on nonconsecutive days (Monday, Wednesday, Friday, or Tuesday, Thursday, and Saturday). These workouts are all you need to activate the powerful fat-mobilizing catecholamines and burn off belly fat in a way that's far more effective than working out every single day. Plus, because of the intense nature of your workout, you need a day off in between workouts. If you're working as hard as you should be during these 28 minutes, three times a week, your body will need time to recover. Remember that muscle is built when you're resting, not when you're working out.

## Be active on rest days

I want to be clear that I'm not suggesting that you should do this routine and then settle into your sofa until the next workout time rolls around. Before obesity and being overweight were an issue for us humans, we walked about 10 miles per day—that was the status quo! While I'm not suggesting that you block out three hours a day to stroll, I am suggesting that you move more and sit less. It's good for your circulation, stabilizes your mood, helps reduce cravings, and increases impulse control. On page 133 in this chapter, you'll find several suggestions for what to do on your active rest days to keep your mind and body feeling it's best.

## What you'll need for the Tiny and Full™ workouts

Make sure you are set up with the following:

- Good fitness shoes
- A room with space to move
- Your favorite music
- Your favorite fitness tracker (mine is the Apple Watch)

## Warming up and cooling down

Before and after every workout, take a few minutes to move your body around to get it ready for your workout and to transition back down when you are done. Walk in place, jog gently, circle your arms, lift and lower your shoulders, lift and lower your knees, or dance around—any sort of movement will do.

## Let's start!

I have outlined 9 different workouts that you will use for the 12 weeks. There is a calendar that organizes the workouts so you'll know exactly what to do each week. Remember, each workout consists of 2 cycles of 4 moves.

Here's how each workout should play out:

**Warm Up**

**Cycle 1**
**Rest 30–60 seconds**

**Cycle 2**
**Rest 30–60 seconds**

**Cycle 1**
**Rest 30–60 seconds**

**Cycle 2**
**Rest 30–60 seconds**

**Cool Down**

**It's time to get your move on!**

## Cycle 1

### Jump Rope
100 reps

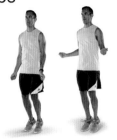

Stand up straight with a slight bend in your knees and hands by your sides. Pretend you're holding a jump rope, and make small circle movements with your hands while quickly jumping up and down on your toes, as you would if you were using a real jump rope.

### Side-to side lunge
30 reps (15 per side)

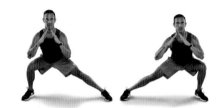

Stand with your feet hip-width apart. Take a giant step out to your right with your right leg and bend your knee to a 90-degree angle. You want to land with your heel first, followed by your forefoot. Press into your foot to return to starting position.

### Power Punch
60 reps
(30 per side)

Stand with feet shoulder-width apart, and right leg slightly in front of the left. Raise your fists up and keep your elbows in and pointing down. Punch your left fist out and across your body, while rotating your torso. Keep your chest lifted. Switch arm and leg stance after 10 punches. Punch as fast and furiously as you can.

### Hip hinger
20 reps

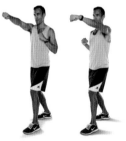

Stand with your feet shoulder-width apart. Shift your weight to your heels and push your hips back as you hinge forward at the hips, keeping your knees slightly bent, until your torso is at about a 45-degree angle. Keep your head, neck, shoulders, chest, and torso in one line, abs engaged and tight. Contract your butt muscles as you lift back up from your hips. Repeat.

## Cycle 2

### High knees
50 reps

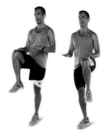

Stand with your feet hip-width apart, chest lifted, shoulders back and down. Place your hands out in front of you with your arms bent at 90 degrees. Drive your right knee toward your chest and quickly place it back on the ground. Immediately drive your left knee toward your chest. Continue alternating quickly.

### Wide squats
15 reps

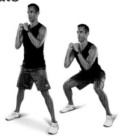

Stand with your feet wider than shoulder width. "Sit down," pushing your buttocks back and keeping your chest up, until your thighs are parallel to the floor. Make sure your knees stay behind your toes. Pause for a second, and then stand up quickly. Repeat, and try to get lower with each squat.

### Side steps
30 reps
(15 per side)

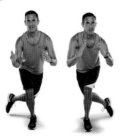

Start off with your feet shoulder-width apart, and body lowered as if you're doing a slight squat. Stay at this height during the entire move (instead of popping up and down). Shuffle feet from side to side by taking one foot out and putting all of your weight on it. Step back and then take the other foot out. Alternate legs.

### Russian twists
30 reps (15 per side)

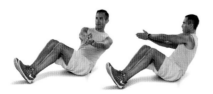

Sit with knees bent and feet together on the floor. Keeping your head, shoulders, and chest all in one line, engage your abs and lean back about 45 degrees, lifting your feet a few inches off the floor. Twist your torso and arms as one unit from side to side, keeping your abdominal muscles engaged. Continue moving side to side.

**Cycle 1**

## Bicycle

40 reps

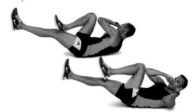

Lie down on your back with knees in toward your chest and hands behind your head. Bring your right elbow toward the left knee while right leg straightens. Alternate sides just like you're pedaling on a bike. Move as quickly as possible, making sure to keep abs braced and tight throughout the movement.

## Plank row

1 minute

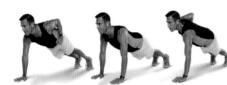

Start in push-up position. Draw right elbow up so that hand comes to rib cage. Lower to starting position, and repeat on left side. Alternate sides, dropping to knees when necessary.

## Slalom

40 reps
(20 per side)

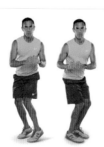

Start with both feet together and your hands in front of you (elbows at your side), as if you're holding ski poles. Jump and twist your upper body in the right and your feet to the left. Then jump up and twist your upper body to the left and your feet to the right. Repeat.

## Military press

30 reps

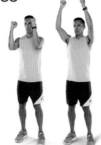

Stand with your feet shoulder-width apart. Make fists and put your elbows at 90 degrees. Raise your arms up above your head. Lower your arms back to 90 degrees. Repeat.

## Cycle 2

### Cross jacks
30 reps

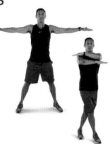

Stand tall with your feet shoulder-width apart and extend your arms straight out to either side with palms facing down. Jump and cross your right arm over your left and your right foot over your left. Jump back to the starting position, then cross with the opposite arm and foot. Continue alternating sides without rest.

### Deep overhead squat
30 reps

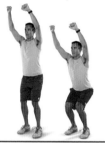

Stand with your feet shoulder-width apart and hands above your head. Bend your knees and squat. Repeat. Keep your hands above your head the whole time.

### Running in place
1 minute

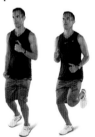

Start jogging in place as fast as you can. Lift your knees up to increase intensity— your thighs can go as high as being parallel to the ground. Remember to move your arms back and forth to boost your heart rate even more. Keep your chest lifted and your head and neck in line with your shoulders.

### Squats
20 reps

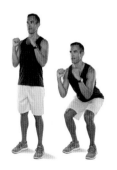

Stand with your feet shoulder-width apart, toes pointed out slightly. Bend your knees to sit back, lowering yourself until your thighs are parallel to the floor. Make sure that your knees stay behind your toes, and keep your chest lifted and your head in line with your neck and shoulders. Pause for a second, and then stand back up to starting position. Repeat.

## Cycle 1

### Side steps
30 reps
(15 per side)

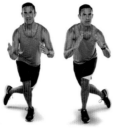

Start off with your feet shoulder-width apart, body lowered as if you're doing a slight squat. Stay at this height during the entire move (instead of popping up and down). Shuffle feet from side to side by taking one foot out and putting all of your weight on it. Step back and then take the other foot out. Alternate legs.

### Curtsey lunge
20 (10 per side)

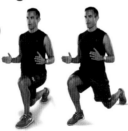

Stand with feet hip-width apart. Take a giant step with your left leg and cross it behind your right. Bend your knees until your right thigh is nearly parallel to the floor. Make sure that your front knee doesn't jut out over your front toes. Press back up to starting position. Step back with other leg. Alternate sides.

### Walking lunges
30 reps
(15 per side)

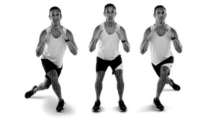

Stand with feet together. Take a giant step forward with your right foot and align knee over ankle. Bend your back knee down close to the floor, heel lifted. Before your back knee touches the floor, push up with your back left leg, \simultaneously bringing your left foot together with your right. Alternate sides without pausing.

### Push-up to knee tuck
10 reps (5 per side)

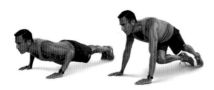

Start in standard push-up position. As you lower your body, bring your right knee up into a tucked position. As you raise your body, bring the leg back out so it's straight and toes are on floor again. Alternate sides.

### Power punch

60 reps
(30 per side)

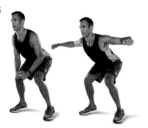

Stand with feet shoulder-width apart, and right leg slightly in front of the left. Raise your fists up and keep your elbows in. Punch your left fist out and across your body, while rotating your torso. Keep your chest lifted and abs tight. Switch arm and leg stance after 10 punches. Punch as fast and furiously as you can.

### Bent over lateral raise

15 reps

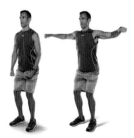

Stand with your legs shoulder-width apart and your knees slightly bent. Lean forward from your hips, keeping your head in line with your shoulders. Let your arms hang. Begin to raise arms to a horizontal position. Pause and contract the shoulder and back muscles. Return to starting position. Repeat.

### Lateral shoulder raises

20 reps

Stand with your feet shoulder-width apart and arms at your side.  With your back straight, raise arms out to shoulder-height with elbows leading the movement. Stop lifting when your arms are at shoulder height. Your upper body should resemble a T. Lower arms toward the starting position in a slow and controlled manner.

### Side-to-side lunge

30 reps (15 per side)

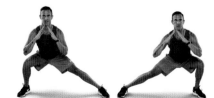

Stand with your feet hip-width apart. Take a giant step out to your right with your right leg and bend your knee to a 90-degree angle. You want to land with your heel first, followed by your forefoot. Press into your foot to return to starting position.

## Cycle 1

### Lateral shuffle
50 reps

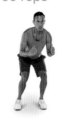
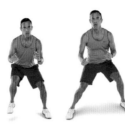

Stand with feet a little wider than hip-distance apart. Shuffle sideways to the right pretending that you are stepping into a ladder on the floor. Step both feet into the first square of the ladder, staying on the balls of your feet. Move your arms to mimic a running motion. After 4 seconds, switch directions and shuffle to the left.

### Plank row
1 minute

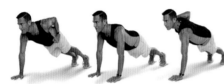

Start in push-up position. Draw right elbow up so that hand comes to rib cage. Lower to starting position, and repeat on left side. Alternate sides, dropping to knees when necessary.

### Jump and butt kick
20 reps

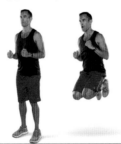

Start by standing up tall. Jump up as high as you can and kick your heels back to your butt so that the two make contact. Land on both feet. Jump back up into the same movement immediately after hitting the ground.

### Lateral shoulder raises
20 reps

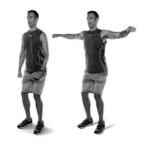

Stand with your feet shoulder-width apart and arms at your side. With your back straight, raise arms out to shoulder-height with elbows leading the movement. Stop lifting when your arms are at shoulder height. Your upper body should resemble a T. Lower arms toward the starting position in a slow and controlled manner.

## Ski jumps

24 reps
(12 per side)

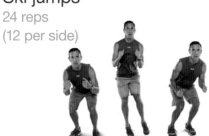

Stand with feet slightly apart, elbows bent as if you were holding ski poles. Jump to the right with both feet. Without pausing, jump back to starting position, and immediately jump again, this time to the other side. Continue alternating, swinging your elbows back and forth to help with your momentum. Keep your chest lifted.

## Russian twists

30 reps (15 per side)

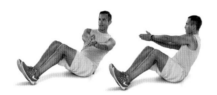

Sit with knees bent and feet together on the floor. Keeping your head, shoulders, and chest all in one line, engage your abs and lean back about 45 degrees, lifting your feet a few inches off the floor. Twist your torso and arms as one unit from side to side, keeping your abdominal muscles engaged. Continue moving side to side.

## Burpees

15 reps

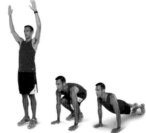

Stand tall with your feet shoulder-width apart. Squat until your hips are lower than your knees. Place your hands on the floor in between your feet and jump your feet back so you're in a push-up position. Jump your feet back up to your hands and stand up tall, finishing by tensing your butt. Repeat.

## Deep overhead squat

30 reps

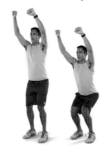

Stand with your feet shoulder-width apart and hands above your head. Bend your knees and squat. Repeat. Keep your hands above your head the whole time.

# Workout 5

## Cycle 1

### Wall sit
1 minute

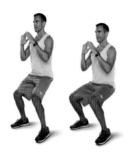

Stand about 2 feet in front of a wall, and lean against it. Slide down until your knees are at 90-degree angles and hold, keeping the abs contracted, for a full minute.

### Squats
20 reps

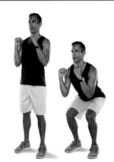

Stand with your feet shoulder-width apart. Bend your knees to sit back, lowering yourself until your thighs are parallel to the floor. Make sure that your knees stay behind your toes, and keep your chest lifted. Pause for a second, and then stand back up to starting position. Repeat.

### Curtsey lunge
20 (10 per side)

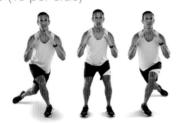

Stand with feet hip-width apart. Take a giant step with your left leg and cross it behind your right. Bend your knees until your right thigh is nearly parallel to the floor. Make sure that your front knee doesn't jut out over your front toes. Press back up to starting position. Step back with other leg. Alternate sides.

### Knee kicks
40 reps
(20 per side)

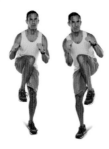

Stand tall with knees slightly bent and fists staggered in front of your face. Drive your right knee up as high as you can and then kick the leg out, extending from the knee out. Add a hop to the movement so that you're jumping each time you raise your knee. Alternate legs. Do not lower arms or rest between kicks.

**Cycle 2**

## Shoulder bridges
30 reps

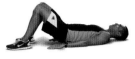
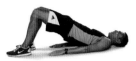

Lie on your back with your knees bent, feet flat on the floor. Lean into your hands and lift your hips, rolling your feet so that they are fl at on the ground. Your body should form a straight line and your arms should be directly below your shoulders. Hold for a count of 2 and gently drop your hips. Repeat.

## Crab kicks
20 reps (10 per side)

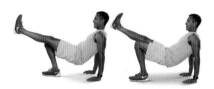

Sit on the floor with the bottom of your feet flat on the floor. Place your hands about one foot behind you, palms flat. Make sure your chest is lifted. Lean into your hands and lift your butt off the floor. Kick right leg up and then lower. Repeat with left. Alternate legs with no rest in between kicks.

## Jump rope
100 reps

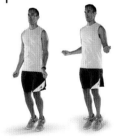

Stand up straight with a slight bend in your knees and hands by your sides. Pretend you're holding a jump rope, and make small circle movements with your hands while quickly jumping up and down on your toes, as you would if you were using a real jump rope.

## Wide squats
15 reps

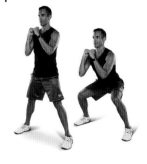

Stand with your feet wider than shoulder width and toes slightly pointed out. "Sit down," pushing your buttocks back and keeping your chest up, until your thighs are parallel to the floor. Look straight ahead, and make sure your knees stay behind your toes. Pause for a second, and then stand up quickly. Repeat, and try to get lower with each squat.

**Cycle 1**

### High Knees
50 reps

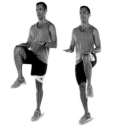

Stand with your feet hip-width apart, chest lifted, and look straight ahead. Place your hands out in front of you with your arms bent at 90 degrees. Drive your right knee toward your chest and quickly place it back on the ground. Immediately drive your left knee toward your chest. Continue alternating knees quickly.

### Hip hinger
20 reps

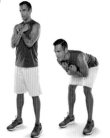

Stand with your feet shoulder-width apart. Shift your weight to your heels and push your hips back as you hinge forward at the hips, until your torso is at about a 45-degree angle. Keep your head, neck, and torso in one line, abs engaged and tight. Contract your butt muscles as you lift back up from your hips. Repeat.

### Butt kicks
60 reps

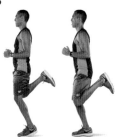

Standing with feet in line with your hips, chest lifted, and looking straight ahead, begin to jog, kicking up your heels behind you. Let your arms move naturally, as they do when you are running. Really exaggerate your back stride, bringing your heels up to your butt. Continue alternating your legs quickly.

### Standing leg raise
40 reps
(20 per side)

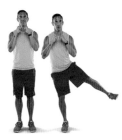

Stand with feet together. If need be, place one hand on the back of a chair to help you balance. Keeping your right leg on the floor, lift your left leg out to the side as high as you can manage. Keep your extended leg straight. Hold this position for a count of 6, and then lower your leg back to the starting position. Now repeat on the opposite side.

## Cycle 2

### Burpees
15 reps

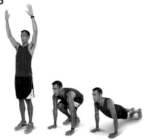

Stand tall with your feet shoulder-width apart. Squat until your hips are lower than your knees. Place your hands on the floor in between your feet and jump your feet back so you're in a push-up position. Jump your feet back up to your hands and stand up tall, finishing by tensing your butt. Repeat.

### Wall sit
1 minute

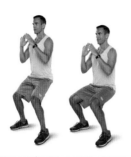

Stand about 2 feet in front of a wall, and lean against it. Slide down until your knees are at 90-degree angles and hold, keeping the abs contracted, for a full minute.

### Slalom
40 reps
(20 per side)

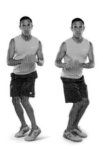

Start with both feet together and your hands in front of you (elbows at your side), as if you're holding ski poles. Jump and twist your upper body in the right and your feet to the left. Then jump up and twist your upper body to the left and your feet to the right. Repeat.

### Frog push-ups
15 reps

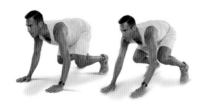

Start in normal push-up position with hands directly under shoulders and fingers pointing forward. Bend your knees at a 90-degree angle and move them in closer to your hands. Bend your elbows and shift your weight forward. Lower your upper body down until your nose is close to the ground, then push back up.

## Cycle 1

### Ski jumps
24 reps
(12 per side)

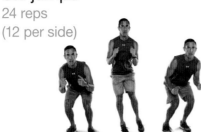

Stand with feet slightly apart, elbows bent as if you were holding ski poles. Jump to the right with both feet. Without pausing, jump back to starting position, and immediately jump again, this time to the other side. Continue alternating, swinging your elbows back and forth to help with your momentum. Keep your chest lifted.

### Shoulder bridges
30 reps

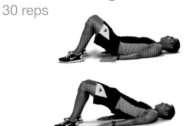

Lie on your back with your knees bent, feet flat on the floor. Lean into your hands and lift your hips, rolling your feet so that they are fl at on the ground. Your body should form a straight line and your arms should be directly below your shoulders. Hold for a count of 2 and gently drop your hips. Repeat.

### Bicycle
40 reps

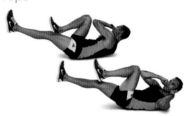

Lie down on your back with knees in toward your chest and hands behind your head. Bring your right elbow toward the left knee while right leg straightens. Alternate sides just like you're pedaling on a bike. Move as quickly as possible, making sure to keep abs braced and tight throughout the movement.

### Power lunges
20 reps

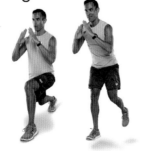

Stand with your feet together and hands on your hips. Bend your knees and hop your feet apart, landing with your right foot forward and your left foot back, knees bent, in a lowered lunge position. Press into your feet and jump back into the air, switching sides. Continue, alternating sides.

### Running in place
1 minute

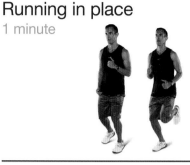

Start jogging in place as fast as you can. Lift your knees up to increase intensity—your thighs can go as high as being parallel to the ground. Remember to move your arms back and forth to boost your heart rate even more. Keep your chest lifted to keep your head and neck in line with your shoulders.

### One-legged Romanian deadlift 20 reps (10 per side)

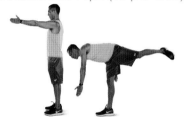

Stand with feet together and arms straight out. Lift leg back slightly so foot is just off floor. Lower your hands to floor while raising lifted leg back behind. Keep your back straight and the knee of supporting leg slightly bent. Once stretch is felt, raise torso and drop leg to return to starting position. Repeat.

### Mountain climbers
40 reps

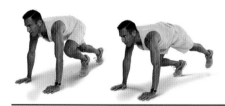

Start in push-up position on hands and toes. Keeping your hips low and your head in line with your spine, bring one knee toward chest and back, and then the other in a fluid motion. Returning each foot to the starting position each time. Alternate sides as quickly as possible.

### Military press
30 reps

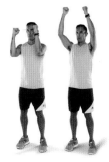

Stand with your feet shoulder-width apart. Make fists and put your elbows at 90 degrees. Raise your arms up above your head. Lower your arms back to 90 degrees. Repeat.

127

## Cycle 1

### Burpees

15 reps

Stand tall with your feet shoulder-width apart. Squat until your hips are lower than your knees. Place your hands on the floor in between your feet and jump your feet back so you're in a push-up position. Jump your feet back up to your hands and stand up tall, finishing by tensing your butt. Repeat.

### Walking lunges

30 reps
(15 per side)

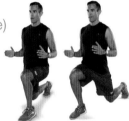

Stand with feet together. Take a giant step forward with your right foot and align knee over ankle. Bend your back knee down close to the floor, heel lifted. Before your back knee touches the floor, push up with your back left leg, simultaneously bringing your left foot together with your right. Alternate sides without pausing.

### Knee kicks

40 reps
(20 per side)

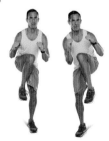

Stand tall with knees slightly bent and fists staggered in front of your face. Drive your right knee up as high as you can and then kick the leg out, extending from the knee out. Add a hop to the movement so that you're jumping each time you raise your knee. Alternate legs. Do not rest between kicks.

### Bent over lateral raise

15 reps

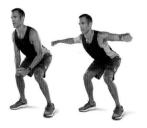

Stand with your legs shoulder-width apart and your knees slightly bent. Lean forward from your hips, keep your back straight, and keep your head in line with your shoulders. Let your arms hang. Begin to raise arms to a horizontal position. Pause and contract the shoulder and back muscles. Return to starting position. Repeat.

## Lateral shuffle

50 reps

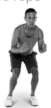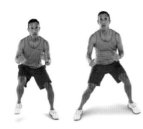

Stand with feet a little wider than hip-distance apart. Shuffle sideways to the right pretending that you are stepping into a ladder on the floor. Step both feet into the first square of the ladder, staying on the balls of your feet. Move your arms to mimic a running motion. After 4 seconds, switch directions and shuffle to the left.

## Standing leg raise

40 reps
(20 per side)

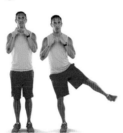

Stand with feet together. Keeping your right leg on the floor, lift your left leg out to the side as high as you can manage. Keep your extended leg straight. Hold this position for a count of 6, and then lower your leg back to the starting position. Now repeat on the opposite side.

## Cross jacks

30 reps

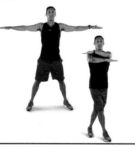

Stand tall with your feet shoulder-width apart and extend your arms straight out to either side with palms facing down. Jump and cross your right arm over your left and your right foot over your left. Jump back to the starting position, then cross with the opposite arm and foot. Continue alternating sides without rest.

## Side lift and lunge

20 reps (10 per side)

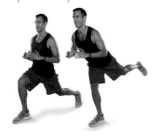

Stand with your feet hip-width apart. Do a side lunge to the right, and at the same time, punch your left hand down toward the floor. Return to standing position and raise both arms directly in front of you to shoulder level (so they're parallel with the floor). At the same time, slightly kick your right leg back. Alternate sides.

## Cycle 1

### Butt kicks
60 reps

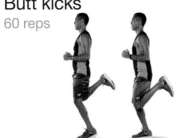

Standing with feet in line with your hips, chest lifted, begin to jog, kicking up your heels behind you. Let your arms move naturally, as they do when you are running. Exaggerate your back stride, bringing your heels up to your butt in an attempt to make contact between the two. Continue alternating your legs quickly.

### Frog push-ups
15 reps

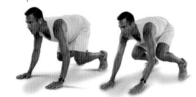

Start in normal push-up position with hands directly under shoulders and fingers pointing forward. Bend your knees at a 90-degree angle and move them in closer to your hands. Bend your elbows and shift your weight forward. Lower your upper body down until your nose is close to the ground, then push back up.

### Mountain climbers
40 reps

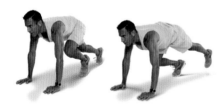

Start in push-up position on hands and toes. Keeping your hips low and your head in line with your spine, bring one knee toward chest and back, and then the other in a fluid motion. Returning each foot to the starting position each time. Alternate sides as quickly as possible.

### One-legged Romanian deadlift 20 reps (10 per side)

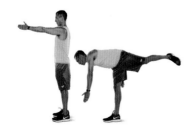

Stand with feet together and arms straight out. Lift leg back slightly so foot is just off floor. Lower your hands to floor while raising lifted leg back behind. Keep your back straight and the knee of supporting leg slightly bent. Once stretch is felt or your hands contacts floor, raise torso and drop leg to return to starting position. Repeat.

Tiny and Full

### Crab kicks
20 (10 per side)

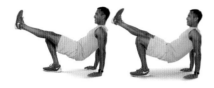

Sit with the bottom of your feet flat on the floor. Place your hands about one foot behind you, palms flat. Make sure your chest is lifted. Lean into your hands and lift your butt off the floor. Kick right leg up and then lower. Repeat with left. Alternate legs with no rest in between kicks.

### Push-up to knee tuck
10 reps (5 per side)

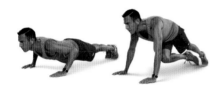

Start in standard push-up position. As you lower your body, bring your right knee up into a tucked position. As you raise your body, bring the leg back out so it's straight and toes are on floor again. Alternate sides.

### Jump and butt kick
20 reps

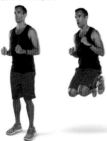

Start by standing up tall. Jump up as high as you can and kick your heels back to your butt so that the two make contact. Land on both feet. Jump back up into the same movement immediately after hitting the ground.

### Power lunges
20 reps

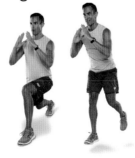

Stand with your feet together and hands on your hips. Bend your knees and hop your feet apart, landing with your right foot forward and your left foot back, knees bent, in a lowered lunge position. Press into your feet and jump back into the air, switching sides. Continue, alternating sides.

# Workout Calendar

## Week 1

Day 1
Workout 1

Day 2
Workout 2

Day 3
Workout 3

## Week 2

Day 1
Workout 1

Day 2
Workout 2

Day 3
Workout 3

## Week 3

Day 1
Workout 4

Day 2
Workout 5

Day 3
Workout 6

## Week 4

Day 1
Workout 4

Day 2
Workout 5

Day 3
Workout 6

## Week 5

Day 1
Workout 1

Day 2
Workout 4

Day 3
Workout 2

## Week 6

Day 1
Workout 1

Day 2
Workout 4

Day 3
Workout 2

## Week 7

Day 1
Workout 5

Day 2
Workout 3

Day 3
Workout 6

## Week 8

Day 1
Workout 5

Day 2
Workout 3

Day 3
Workout 6

## Week 9

Day 1
Workout 4

Day 2
Workout 7

Day 3
Workout 5

## Week 10

Day 1
Workout 4

Day 2
Workout 7

Day 3
Workout 5

## Week 11

Day 1
Workout 7

Day 2
Workout 8

Day 3
Workout 9

## Week 12

Day 1
Workout 7

Day 2
Workout 8

Day 3
Workout 9

# What to Do on Your Active Rest Days

There's plenty of science to support that an active lifestyle will benefit your overall health. In fact, in a giant survey that followed the exercise habits and quality of health in more than 250,000 men and women ages 50 to 71 years old for nearly a decade, researchers found that the people who exercised vigorously for 20 minutes, three times a week were 32 percent less likely to die from any health cause, and people who exercised moderately at least 30 minutes most days of the week were 27 percent less likely to die from any health cause. Put these two together, and you should be living a long healthy and happy life. Can't think of an activity? Try one of the following.

## Go for a walk.

Taking a walk won't impede your body's recovery from your Tiny and Full™ work-outs, and it provides multiple benefits beyond physical health. Some studies have found that walking can counter faltering memories in people over age 50. This makes perfect sense to me because when I walk, I think. It's an easy, natural movement that doesn't really engage our brains, but it does refresh and rejuvenate our minds. So we can reflect on a problem (and a solution) or even meditate in our own way. Consider taking a walk at a local park, at the beach, at a lake, or even in a pretty neighborhood. Research shows that any sort of a "green" or "nature" walk can boost mood, lower anxiety, improve willpower and impulse control, and increase overall energy. Walks are also a great activity to do with someone else because the easy pace lets you carry on a conversation—and the complete lack of distractions provides a focus we don't usually get in our hectic lives.

## Ride a bike.

Leisure bike riding can provide all the benefits you get on a walk. No matter your age or fitness level, you can enjoy the scenery and feel the wind whip through your hair just like when you were a kid. Another benefit of peddling is that it can help keep you feeling happy! In a survey conducted by Portland State University, respondents who biked to work reported the highest levels of well-being.

## Say "Namaste."

A favorite "rest" day activity of one of my clients is yoga, often because it provides a great stretch for hardworking muscles. While flexibility improves, so does strength,

# My Tech Secret to Better Fitness

I am always searching for a smarter way to stay motivated with fitness. My top pick for myself, my family, and all my celebrity clients is the Apple Watch. It is probably the most valuable tool I use daily to track my fitness. If you follow me on Instagram (@JorgeCruise or @TinyandFull), you can probably tell that I always have my watch on. It takes fitness monitoring to a whole new level by encouraging healthier behaviors like sitting less, moving more, and getting brisk exercise.

The secret to the Apple Watch is the Activity App, which is critical in tracking three vital pieces of information. It reminds you to **stand** and allows you to visually see how many hours each day you've been on your feet. The second thing it tracks is when you **move** by showing you how many active calories you've burned throughout the day. Finally, it tracks your **exercise** by monitoring any brisk activity you've done throughout the day, such as the HIIT workouts in this book. It will tell you how many minutes you've done with a goal of 30 per day.

The Apple Watch truly tracks it all! With an emphasis on Stand, Move, and Exercise, you will constantly be reminded to sit less (such as when you're relaxing at the pool), move more (such as by taking a hike), and do 30 minutes of brisk activity (such as HIIT)!

The bottom line is that being more aware is key...and as we all know, knowledge is power. So don't just guess how many calories you've eaten or burned today . . . track them! You will know exactly where you stand with the Apple Watch . . . no pun intended.

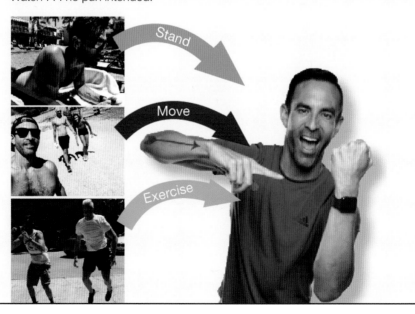

as yoga incorporates movements such as the plank, which not only tones muscles but helps you become stronger. Other yoga benefits are wonderful too, like helping you get a better night's sleep! A study in *Medical Science Monitor* found that patients with sleep problems reported an improved quality of their sleep on days when they did yoga and meditation. Doing yoga also releases feel-good chemicals in your brain. Scientists at Boston University School of Medicine and McLean Hospital were able to see that people who did yoga for 30 minutes had a 27 percent increase of gamma-aminobutyric acid (GABA) in their brains. This feel-good chemical helps regulate nerve activity—it's reduced in people with mood and anxiety disorders, so the goal is to have more if you want to feel happier and more relaxed.

## Take a hike.

Most of us live within driving distance to some truly beautiful nature. Get up close and personal with all of nature's splendor by taking a hike. It's one of my favorite ways to leave behind the hustle, bustle, and fast pace of everyday life. Make sure to take along your smartphone, not just to snap photos, but to make the most out of some helpful hiking apps, such as The Spot, a free GPS tracker that uploads real-time information on your location and condition. Bring a friend along too, especially if you're heading somewhere without a lot of foot traffic.

## Put on your dancing shoes.

You can always just rock out at home to your favorite music, or take a jazz, tap, or hip-hop class at a local community college; many gyms also have Zumba. Or, if you have a willing partner, sign up for ballroom dance classes, or check out your local churches and community centers for line dancing, square dancing, contra dancing, salsa, or Zydeco dancing. Nobody to go with you? No problem. Many of the just-mentioned classes offer singles options, so just ask. This is a great way to get some social—or one-on-one—time and do it while moving your body. Besides being a fun activity on your "rest" days, I absolutely love this idea for date night— instead of going out for a heavy dinner and a movie, you can have a light dinner and get your move on.

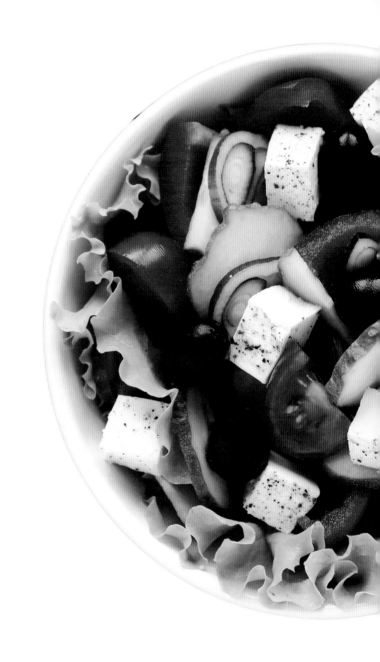

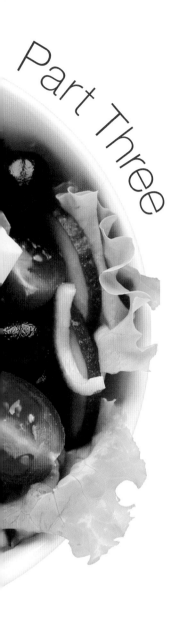

# Part Three

# Tiny and Full™ Forever

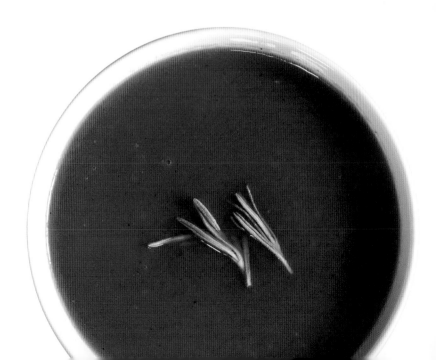

# 6 Beyond the 12 Weeks

You did it!

If you are reading this chapter, you have hopefully completed the 12-week challenge. Congrats! If you are looking ahead and have yet to finish—or even start—the 12 weeks, that's okay! It's good to be prepared.

So here's what to do now that the initial 12 weeks are over. As you have been doing each week, it's time to take an "after" photo to capture your complete transformation. You will appreciate this in the months to come. I challenge you to share this photo with me and others. Visit Tiny and Full™ on Facebook, Instagram, or Twitter to share your story with me.

Now, you have a few options on how to proceed. Choose one of following option paths to make this a sustainable lifestyle.

## OPTION 1: Keep it simple.

Repeat this book. Simply return to the meal planners and workouts and keep following them. There is power in simplicity, and automation is the key to success. This option is great for those of you who enjoy a done-for-you, laid out plan that requires no thinking.

## OPTION 2: Step out on your own.

If you are comfortable with the tools I have provided in this book but don't want to follow the meal planners or workouts again, feel free to step out on your own. You can use the food list in Chapter 7 to make your own menus. Use the recipes and meal planners as structure and inspiration. Just keep in mind your calorie goal and plan ahead. It's never any fun to get to dinner and realize you've eaten most of your calories. Planning ahead is key! You can also use the exercises found in Chapter 5 and mix and match the cycles to make your own workouts.

Quick tips for stepping out on your own:

- Use the food list.

- Use recipes and meal planners for ideas.

- Stick to Level 1 foods as much as possible. Make them the majority of your meal.

- Think of Level 2–4 foods as condiments.

- Use the workouts for ideas to create your own cycles.

## OPTION 3: Let me help.

Visit TinyandFull.com for online coaching and direct support from me, as well as new meal planners, recipes, and my fit kits for maximum workout results and variety. You can also check out Tiny and Full™ on social media for inspiration, tips, recipes, and more.

Facebook.com/TinyandFull

Instagram/TinyandFull

Twitter/TinyandFull

#TinyandFull

So now you have the information you need to take this book beyond the 12 weeks and make it a sustainable routine. Remember to keep me updated on your progress and success, as well as get tips, recipes, and inspiration, by following Tiny and Full™ on Facebook, Instagram, and Twitter!

## What to do when you reach your goal weight

When you reach your goal, feel free to switch to 1,800 or even 2,000 calories a day. Keep monitoring your weight and adjust accordingly.

# 7 Tiny and Full™ Foods

The following list of foods will help you if you are stepping out on your own and want to make your own meals and menu planners.

The foods are organized alphabetically according to food categories. The four levels are color-coded to help you easily identify foods that are lowest in calorie density, as shown in the following legend:

Level 1: Minimal Calorie Density

Level 2: Low Calorie Density

Level 3: Medium Calorie Density

Level 4: High Calorie Density

Remember, when making meals, you want to make the majority of your meal come from Level 1 foods. Dip into Level 2 occasionally, watch your portions of Level 3, and try to minimize or avoid Level 4. Levels 2–4 are to be thought of as condiments to Level 1. You will notice that oils, such as olive oil, are a Level 4. While we definitely want to minimize the usage of oils due to their low calorie density, oils do help with cooking and baking. Just remember to use them in small amounts (check out the recipes in Chapter 8 for examples). Other Level 4 items, such as sugary snacks and treats, should be avoided.

Each food on the list will show you two things: the calorie density number and a real-life conversion. This real-life conversion will show you what 100 calories of that particular food looks like. For example, the energy density of watermelon (Level 1) is .26. But what does that mean? That is where this conversion comes into play to let you know that 100 calories of watermelon is about 2 cups, diced. Compare that to 100 calories of walnuts (Level 4), which is only 7 halves. This is meant to give you a visual example to help you understand what calorie density looks like.

Use this list to help pick lower-calorie-density foods as much as possible. If you want to calculate the calorie density of a food not on this list, simply look at the label and divide the number of calories in the food by the number of grams.

Calorie density = calories ÷ grams

Happy eating!

# Tiny and Full™ Food List

| Calorie Density Legend | |
| --- | --- |
| Level 1: Minimal Calorie Density | From 0–0.59 |
| Level 2: Low Calorie Density | From 0.6–1.5 |
| Level 3: Medium Calorie Density | From 1.6–3.9 |
| Level 4: High Calorie Density | From 4.0–9.0 |

## Fruit

| | Calorie Density | Real-Life Conversion |
| --- | --- | --- |
| Acai berries, dried | 0.70 | 5 oz. |
| Apple | 0.56 | 1 medium |
| Applesauce, unsweetened | 0.41 | 2 cups |
| Apricot | 0.51 | 6 apricots |

# Fruit (continued)

| | Calorie Density | Real-Life Conversion |
|---|---|---|
| Avocado | 1.90 | ⅓ cup |
| Banana | 0.90 | 1 7-inch banana |
| Banana, dried | 3.71 | 1 oz. |
| Blackberries | 0.60 | 1⅓ cups |
| Blueberries | 0.57 | 1¼ cups |
| Boysenberry | 0.50 | 1½ cups |
| Cantaloupe | 0.34 | 2 cups cubed |
| Cherries | 0.70 | 1 cup |
| Cherry tomatoes | 0.18 | 32 cherry tomatoes |
| Currant | 2.68 | 1.3 oz. |
| Date | 1.17 | 3 dates |
| Date, dried | 3.00 | 1 oz. |
| Dragon fruit | 0.60 | 1¾ dragon fruit |
| Durian | 1.47 | ¼ cup |
| Fig | 0.73 | 2 figs |
| Fig, dried | 2.47 | 2 figs |
| Gogi berry, dried | .3.21 | ¼ cup |
| Grape | 0.41 | 62 grapes |
| Guava | 0.68 | 2 medium |
| Honeydew | 0.33 | ¼ 5-inch melon |
| Kiwi | 0.61 | 2 large |
| Kirkland Frozen Blueberries | 0.50 | 1 cup |
| Kirkland Frozen Strawberries | 0.36 | 2 cups |
| Kumquat | 0.68 | 7 kumquats |
| Lemon | 0.29 | 5 lemons |
| Lime | 0.30 | 5 limes |
| Loquat | 0.47 | 11 large |
| Mango | 0.60 | ⅔ medium |
| Mulberry | 0.43 | 1½ cups |
| Nectarine | 0.64 | 1½ large nectarines |
| Olive | 1.14 | 18 olives |

## Fruit (continued)

| | Calorie Density | Real-Life Conversion |
|---|---|---|
| Orange | 0.47 | 1¼ large orange |
| Papaya | 0.43 | ½ medium papaya |
| Passion fruit | 0.97 | 5 passion fruits |
| Peach | 0.50 | 2½ medium peaches |
| Pear | 0.51 | 1 medium pear |
| Persimmon, Japanese | 0.70 | ¾ whole persimmon |
| Pineapple | 0.56 | 1¼ cups of chunks |
| Plum | 0.60 | 3 medium plums |
| Plum tomato | 0.17 | 9 and ½ plum tomatoes |
| Plum, prune | 2.40 | 5 prunes |
| Pomegranate | 0.83 | 1 medium pomegranate |
| Pumpkin | 0.20 | 2 cups mashed |
| Raisin | 3.25 | 2 miniature boxes |
| Raspberry | 0.57 | 1½ cups |
| Red and pink grapefruit | 0.42 | 1 4-inch grapefruit |
| Squash, all | 0.20 | 3 cups sliced |
| Star fruit | 0.31 | 2½ star fruits |
| Strawberry | 0.32 | 25 medium |
| Tamarillo | 0.33 | 5 tamarillos |
| Tiny and Full™ Power Fruits, with 8 oz. water | 0.13 | 3 fruits and a 3-oz. shake |
| Tomato | 0.17 | 4¾ medium tomatoes |
| Watermelon | 0.26 | 2 cups diced |

## Vegetables

| | Calorie Density | Real-Life Conversion |
|---|---|---|
| Alfalfa spouts | 0.20 | 13 cups |
| Artichoke | 0.53 | 1½ medium artichokes |
| Arugula | 0.25 | 20 cups |
| Asparagus | 0.22 | 30 spears ½-inch base |
| Bell pepper | 0.20 | 5 medium bell peppers |

# My Go-To List for Costco

In order to save time and money, I am a Costco member. I love their Kirkland Signature brand foods for their quality and pricing.

Below is my go-to shopping list of my favorite kind of *Kirkland Signature* items that I always grab when I am at Costco. Check out the food list for their calorie density values.

Make sure to check out Costco.com for more Kirkland Signature products as well as follow Costco on Facebook (www.facebook.com/Costco) and Instagram (@Costco).

☐ Greek Yogurt

☐ Chicken Breast

☐ Rotisserie Chicken

☐ Sockeye Salmon Fillets

☐ Lean Ground Beef

☐ Chocolate Chip Oatmeal

☐ Cooked Quinoa

☐ Basmati Rice

☐ Multigrain Whole Wheat Grain Bread

☐ Frozen Strawberries

☐ Frozen Green Beans

☐ Frozen Mixed Vegetables

☐ Frozen Blueberries

☐ Unsweetened Tea

☐ Coffee Sumatra

☐ Coffee Costa Rica

☐ Coffee Guatemalan Lake Atitlan

☐ Coffee Rwanda

☐ Coffee Panama Geisha

☐ Bottled Water

Tiny and Full™ Foods

# Vegetables (continued)

| | Calorie Density | Real-Life Conversion |
|---|---|---|
| Bok choy | 0.14 | 10 cups |
| Broccoli | 0.35 | 3 cups chopped |
| Brussels sprouts | 0.36 | 1¾ cups |
| Cabbage | 0.23 | 4½ cup chopped |
| Carrot | 0.41 | 4 medium |
| Cauliflower | 0.23 | 4 cups |
| Celery | 0.15 | 16½ medium stalks |
| Chard | 0.19 | 14 cups |
| Collard greens | 0.26 | 9 cups |
| Corn, white | 0.86 | ¾ cup |
| Corn, yellow | 0.96 | ¾ cup |
| Cucumber | 0.15 | 6⅓ cups sliced |
| Eggplant | 0.33 | ¾ cup |
| Endive | 0.16 | 12½ cups |
| Fennel | 0.31 | 1⅓ bulb |
| Green bean | 0.35 | 60 beans 4 inches long |
| Green onion | 0.33 | 20 medium 4 inches long |
| Jicama | 0.38 | 2 cups |
| Kale | 0.49 | 13 cups chopped |
| Kirkland Frozen Mixed Vegetables | 0.33 | 2.5 cups |
| Kirkland Green Beans | 0.17 | 2.5 tbsp. |
| Lettuce, iceberg | 0.14 | 11 cups shredded |
| Lettuce, red leaf | 0.16 | 22 cups shredded |
| Lettuce, romaine | 0.17 | 12 cups shredded |
| Mint | 0.43 | 8 oz. |
| Mushroom | 0.26 | 26 medium |
| Mustard green | 0.27 | 7 cups |
| Okra | 0.23 | 2½ cups |
| Onion | 0.43 | 2 medium onions |
| Pepper, jalapeño | 0.29 | 25 peppers |
| Pepper, serrano | 0.33 | 50 peppers |

# Vegetables (continued)

| | Calorie Density | Real-Life Conversion |
|---|---|---|
| Pickle, dill | 0.12 | 6 large pickles |
| Pickles, gherkin | 0.14 | 20 pickles |
| Potato, baked | 0.97 | ¾ small potato |
| Potato, french fries, fast food | 3.07 | ¼ medium order |
| Potato, french fries, home made | 2.67 | ⅔ cup |
| Potato, mashed with whole milk and margarine | 1.13 | ⅔ cup |
| Radicchio | 0.23 | 50 radicchios |
| Radish | 0.11 | 101 radishes |
| Rutabaga, cubed | 0.39 | 2 cups |
| Seaweed, nori | 4.00 | 10 sheets |
| Shallots | 0.70 | 14 tbsp. |
| Spinach | 0.23 | 14 cups |
| Sweet potato, baked | 0.90 | ¾ medium potato |
| Tiny and Full™ Chocolate Pea Protein, with 8 oz. water | 0.21 | 1 protein and a 7-oz. shake |
| Tiny and Full™ Essential Fiber | 4.00 | 10 tsp. |
| Tiny and Full™ Power Greens | 0.15 | 3 shakes |
| Tiny and Full™ Unflavored Pea Protein, with 8 oz. water | 0.22 | 1 protein and a 6-oz. shake |
| Tiny and Full™ Vanilla Pea Protein, with 8 oz. water | 0.21 | 1 protein and a 7-oz. shake |
| Turnip greens | 0.20 | 5 cups |
| Turnip, cubed | 0.22 | 3 cups |
| Vegetable blend, stir fry frozen | 0.25 | 2½ cups |
| Watercress | 0.20 | 20 cups chopped |

# Legumes

| | Calorie Density | Real-Life Conversion |
|---|---|---|
| Baked beans, original, Bush's Best | 1.19 | ⅓ cup |
| Black beans, cooked | 1.32 | ⅓ cup |
| Chickpeas | 1.19 | ⅓ cup |

## Legumes (continued)

| | Calorie Density | Real-Life Conversion |
|---|---|---|
| Edamame, shelled | 1.60 | ⅓ cup |
| Hummus | 1.80 | 4 tbsp. |
| Kidney beans | 1.27 | ⅓ cup |
| Lentils | 1.14 | ⅓ cup |
| Peanut butter | 5.88 | 1 tbsp. |
| Pinto beans | 1.43 | ⅓ cup |

## Pasta

| | Calorie Density | Real-Life Conversion |
|---|---|---|
| Brown rice pasta, any size, cooked | 1.23 | ⅓ cup |
| Gluten-free pasta, any size, cooked | 1.31 | ⅓ cup |
| Traditional, any size, cooked | 1.58 | ⅓ cup |
| Whole-wheat, any size, cooked | 1.24 | ½ cup |

## Fish & Seafood

| | Calorie Density | Real-Life Conversion |
|---|---|---|
| Catfish | 1.35 | 2½ oz. |
| Clams | 1.48 | 2⅓ oz. |
| Cod | 1.05 | 3⅓ oz. |
| Crab | 1.11 | 3 oz. |
| Flounder | 0.91 | 3¾ oz. |
| Halibut | 0.94 | 3¾ oz. |
| Kirkland Sockeye Salmon Fillets | 1.59 | 2.2 oz. |
| Lobster | 0.90 | 3¾ oz. |
| Mahi mahi | 1.09 | 3¼ oz. |
| Orange roughy | 1.05 | 3⅓ oz. |
| Oysters | 0.51 | 14 medium |
| Salmon | 1.32 | 2½ oz. |
| Sardines | 1.64 | 2 oz. |
| Scallops | 0.87 | 8 large or 20 small |

# Fish & Seafood (continued)

| | Calorie Density | Real-Life Conversion |
|---|---|---|
| Shrimp | 1.18 | 3 oz. |
| Sole | 1.05 | 3⅓ oz. |
| Swordfish | 1.55 | 2¼ oz. |
| Tilapia | 0.96 | 3½ oz. |
| Trout | 1.50 | 2⅓ oz. |
| Tuna, canned | 1.16 | 3 oz. |
| Tuna, fresh | 1.39 | 2½ oz. |

# Poultry

| | Calorie Density | Real-Life Conversion |
|---|---|---|
| Chicken, breast, without skin | 1.25 | 2¾ oz. |
| Chicken, leg, without skin | 1.91 | 1¾ oz. |
| Chicken, thigh, without skin | 1.41 | 2½ oz. |
| Chicken, wing, without skin | 2.05 | 1¾ oz. |
| Duck, breast, without skin | 1.29 | 2¾ oz. |
| Kirkland Chicken Breast | 0.98 | 1 piece |
| Kirkland Rotisserie Chicken | 1.65 | 2 oz. |
| Processed sandwich/ deli meats – chicken | 1.15 | 3 oz. |
| Processed sandwich/ deli meats – turkey | 1.13 | 3 oz. |
| Sausage, chicken | 2.12 | ⅔ link |
| Sausage, turkey | 1.61 | ¾ link |
| Turkey bacon | 1.29 | 2¾ oz. |
| Turkey bacon, lean | 1.29 | 2¾ oz. |
| Turkey breast | 2.33 | 1½ oz. |
| Turkey burger | 1.34 | 2½ oz. |
| Turkey leg with skin | 2.08 | 1¾ oz. |
| Turkey thigh | 1.25 | 2¾ oz. |
| Turkey, lean ground, 85% fat-free | 2.14 | 1½ oz. |
| Turkey, lean ground, 99% fat-free | 1.52 | 2¼ oz. |

# Red Meat & Pork

| | Calorie Density | Real-Life Conversion |
|---|---|---|
| Bacon | 5.42 | 3 slices |
| Beef chuck | 3.45 | 1 oz. |
| Beef flank | 1.94 | 1.8 oz. |
| Beef jerky | 4.10 | 1¼ pieces |
| Beef porterhouse | 2.04 | 1.7 oz. |
| Beef rib | 2.95 | ¼ rib |
| Beef round, sirloin | 1.86 | 1.9 oz. |
| Beef rump roast | 1.92 | 1.8 oz. |
| Beef T-bone steak | 2.21 | 1.6 oz. |
| Beef tenderloin | 2.11 | 1.6 oz. |
| Bison, ground | 2.38 | 1.5 oz. |
| Bologna | 3.11 | 1¼ slices |
| Canadian bacon | 1.37 | 2½ oz. |
| Chorizo, beef | 4.08 | ⅔ link |
| Chorizo, pork | 2.71 | ½ sausage |
| Corned beef | 1.89 | 1.8 oz. |
| Ground beef, 75% fat-free | 2.54 | 1.3 oz. |
| Ground beef, 85% fat-free | 2.27 | 1.5 oz. |
| Ground beef, 95% fat-free | 1.64 | 2.15 oz. |
| Ham, extra lean | 1.07 | 3⅓ oz. |
| Ham, regular | 1.64 | 2 6-inch slices |
| Hot dog | 3.09 | ¾ dog |
| Hot dog, 97% fat-free | 1.01 | 2 dogs |
| Hot dog, vegan | 1.32 | 2 dogs |
| Hot dog, veggie dog | 1.25 | 2 dogs |
| Kirkland 9% Lean Ground Beef | .61 | 2.2 oz. |
| Lamb chop | 2.83 | 1.25 oz. |
| Lamb leg | 2.65 | 1.3 oz. |
| Lamb roast | 2.65 | 1.3 oz. |
| Liverwurst | 3.21 | 1 oz. |
| Pastrami | 1.46 | 2½ oz. |

# Red Meat & Pork (continued)

| | Calorie Density | Real-Life Conversion |
|---|---|---|
| Pastrami, 98% fat-free | 0.95 | 3¾ oz. |
| Pepperoni | 4.91 | 4 × 1³⁄₈ inch diameter slices |
| Pork center loin chop | 2.02 | 1.7 oz. |
| Pork tenderloin | 1.44 | 2½ oz. |
| Processed sandwich/ deli meats – ham | 1.11 | 3 oz. |
| Processed sandwich/ deli meats – roast beef | 1.19 | 3 oz. |
| Prosciutto | 2.25 | 3 slices |
| Roast beef | 1.11 | 3 oz. |
| Salami | 2.61 | 1²⁄₃ slice |
| Sausage, breakfast | 2.42 | 2 4-inch links |
| Sausage, polish | 3.26 | ⅓ link |
| Veal loin chop or roast | 1.75 | 2 oz. |

# Cereals & Grains

| | Calorie Density | Real-Life Conversion |
|---|---|---|
| Basmati rice, cooked | 1.20 | ½ cup |
| Brown rice, cooked | 1.11 | ⅓ cup |
| Cereal, Cheerios | 3.57 | 1 cup |
| Cereal, Ezekiel 4:9 sprouted whole grain | 3.33 | ¼ cup |
| Cereal, Ezekiel 4:9 sprouted whole grain golden flax | 3.15 | ¼ cup |
| Cereal, Post shredded wheat | 3.47 | ⅔ cup |
| Cereal, Total | 3.33 | ¾ cup |
| Cereal, Wheaties | 3.70 | ¾ cup |
| Corn-muffin "Jiffy" | 4.84 | ½ of a small muffin |
| Couscous, cooked | 1.12 | ⅔ cup |
| Croutons | 4.07 | ¾ cup |
| Granola, low-fat without raisins | 3.80 | ¼ cup |
| Jasmine rice, cooked | 1.03 | ½ cup |

Tiny and Full™ Foods

## Cereals & Grains (continued)

| | Calorie Density | Real-Life Conversion |
|---|---|---|
| Oatmeal, instant, apples and cinnamon, cooked | 1.08 | ¼ cup |
| Oatmeal, instant, cooked | 0.91 | ⅓ cup |
| Oatmeal, steel cut, cooked | 0.71 | ⅔ cup |
| Quinoa, cooked | 1.20 | ⅓ cup |
| Spanish rice, cooked | 0.87 | ⅓ cup |
| White rice, cooked | 1.30 | ½ cup |

## Breads & Tortillas

| | Calorie Density | Real-Life Conversion |
|---|---|---|
| Bagels, honey whole-wheat | 3.08 | 1¼ slices |
| Bread, sprouted whole-grain | 2.35 | 1¼ slices |
| Bread, whole-wheat | 2.44 | 1½ slices |
| Hamburger bun | 2.62 | 1 bun |
| Hamburger bun, sprouted whole-grain | 2.44 | ½ bun |
| Kirkland Multigrain 100% Whole Wheat Grain Bread | 2.64 | ⅔ slice |
| Pancakes, plain frozen, ready-to-heat | 2.31 | 1 pancake |
| Pita, whole-wheat | 2.66 | ½ 6-inch pita |
| Roll, dinner | 3.33 | 1 2-inch square roll |
| Tortilla, corn | 2.14 | 2 6-inch tortillas |
| Tortilla, flour | 2.86 | 1 6-inch tortilla |
| Waffles, frozen | 2.00 | 1⅓ waffles |
| Wrap, whole-wheat | 2.86 | 1¼ 6-inch tortillas |

## Dairy

| | Calorie Density | Real-Life Conversion |
|---|---|---|
| Greek yogurt | 0.97 | ½ container |
| Greek yogurt, fruit on the bottom | 0.82 | ⅔ container |
| Greek yogurt, nonfat | 0.57 | 1 container |
| Half-and-half | 1.33 | 5 tbsp. |

## Dairy (continued)

| | Calorie Density | Real-Life Conversion |
|---|---|---|
| Kirkland Greek Yogurt | 0.57 | ¾ cup |
| Milk, 1% | 0.42 | 8 oz. |
| Milk, 2% | 0.50 | 7 oz. |
| Milk, fat-free | 0.35 | 10 oz. |
| Milk, whole | 0.63 | 5 oz. |
| Rice milk, plain | 0.49 | 7 oz. |
| Sour cream | 1.67 | 4 tbsp. |
| Soy milk, plain, Silk | 0.54 | 6 oz. |
| Whipped cream, Cool-Whip | 2.75 | 8 tbsp. |
| Whipped cream, Cool-Whip, fat-free | 1.67 | 13 tbsp. |
| Whipped cream, extra creamy | 4.00 | 10 tbsp. |
| Whipped cream, fat-free | 1.00 | 40 tbsp. |
| Whipping cream | 3.47 | 13 tbsp. |
| Yogurt, fat-free, plain | 0.44 | 8 oz. |
| Yogurt, fat-free, strawberry | 0.44 | 8 oz. |
| Yogurt, plain | 0.61 | ⅔ container |
| Yogurt, strawberry | 0.97 | ½ container |

## Cheese

| | Calorie Density | Real-Life Conversion |
|---|---|---|
| American | 2.38 | 1½ oz. |
| Asiago | 3.57 | 1 oz. |
| Blue | 3.57 | 1 oz. |
| Brick | 3.57 | 1 oz. |
| Brie | 3.35 | 1 oz. |
| Cheddar | 4.04 | ¾ oz. |
| Colby | 3.93 | ¾ oz. |
| Colby Jack | 3.93 | ¾ oz. |
| Cottage cheese, 1% fat | 0.72 | ⅔ cup |
| Cottage cheese, 2% fat | 0.90 | ½ cup |
| Cottage cheese, 4% fat | 0.93 | ⅓ cup |

| | Calorie Density | Real-Life Conversion |
|---|---|---|
| Cottage cheese, fat-free | 0.62 | ²/₃ cup |
| Cream cheese | 2.58 | 1¹/₃ oz. |
| Cream cheese, fat-free | 0.93 | 7 tbsp. |
| Cream cheese, strawberry light | 2.17 | 5 tbsp. |
| Cream cheese, whipped | 2.27 | 4 tbsp. |
| Edam | 3.57 | 1 oz. |
| Farmer cheese | 3.57 | 1 oz. |
| Feta | 2.63 | 1¹/₃ oz. |
| Fontina | 3.89 | ¾ oz. |
| Gorgonzola | 3.36 | 1 oz. |
| Gouda | 3.57 | 1 oz. |
| Gruyère | 4.14 | ¾ oz. |
| Havarti | 3.93 | ¾ oz. |
| Limburger | 3.28 | 1 oz. |
| Mascarpone | 4.64 | ¾ oz. |
| Monterey Jack | 3.71 | 1 oz. |
| Mozzarella, part skim milk | 2.54 | 1¹/₃ oz. |
| Mozzarella, whole milk | 3.00 | 1 oz. |
| Muenster | 3.57 | 1 oz. |
| Parmesan | 3.92 | ¾ oz. |
| Pepper Jack | 3.77 | 1 oz. |
| Provolone | 3.50 | 1 oz. |
| Queso blanco | 3.93 | ¾ oz. |
| Ricotta, part skim milk | 1.38 | ¹/₃ cup |
| Ricotta, whole milk | 1.74 | ¼ cup |
| Romano | 3.89 | ¾ oz. |
| String cheese | 2.86 | 1¼ oz. |
| String cheese, light | 2.38 | 1½ oz. |
| Swiss | 3.79 | 1 oz. |

## Eggs

| | Calorie Density | Real-Life Conversion |
|---|---|---|
| Egg beaters | 0.53 | 6 eggs |
| Egg, white | 0.52 | 6 eggs |
| Egg, whole | 1.44 | 1⅓ eggs |
| Avocado oil | 8.99 | 3 tsp. |

## Fats

| | Calorie Density | Real-Life Conversion |
|---|---|---|
| Barlean's Key Lime Omega Swirl To Go | 6.00 | 1½ tsp. |
| Butter | 7.20 | 1 tbsp. |
| Butter, substitute | 4.93 | 1½ tbsp. |
| Butter, substitute, light | 2.86 | 2½ tbsp. |
| Coconut oil | 8.93 | 3 tsp. |
| Crisco | 9.17 | 3 tsp. |
| Flaxseed oil | 5.87 | 3 tsp. |
| Ghee | 9.00 | 3 tsp. |
| Lard | 8.98 | 3 tsp. |
| Olive oil | 8.00 | 3 tsp. |
| Sesame oil | 8.89 | 3 tsp. |
| Walnut oil | 8.89 | 3 tsp. |

## Nuts* & Seeds

| | Calorie Density | Real-Life Conversion |
|---|---|---|
| Almond butter, unsweetened | 6.15 | 1 tbsp. |
| Almond flour/meal | 5.80 | ⅛ cup |
| Almonds | 5.80 | 15 almonds |
| Brazil nuts | 6.53 | 3 nuts |
| Cashews | 6.28 | 25 halves |
| Coconut, flour | 6.45 | ¼ cup |

*Nuts are shaded in pink because they are energy dense; however, they are very filling and satiating and are generally associated with health benefits and weight control, not weight gain.

## Nuts* & Seeds (continued)

| | Calorie Density | Real-Life Conversion |
|---|---|---|
| Coconut, meat, dried | 6.61 | ½ oz. |
| Coconut, meat, raw | 3.53 | ⅓ cup shredded |
| Coconut, meat, sweetened | 4.56 | ⅕ cup shredded |
| Macadamia nuts | 6.28 | 5 nuts |
| Pecans | 7.00 | 10 pieces |
| Pine nuts | 5.71 | ⅛ cup |
| Pumpkin seeds | 5.60 | 2 tbsp. |
| Sunflower seeds | 5.85 | ⅛ cup without shells |
| Walnuts | 6.54 | 7 halves |

## Herbs & Spices

| | Calorie Density | Real-Life Conversion |
|---|---|---|
| Basil | 0.17 | 1,470 leaves |
| Chives | 0.33 | 100 tbsp. |
| Cilantro | 0.20 | 25 cups |
| Garlic | 1.33 | 25 cloves |
| Ginger | 0.50 | 33 tbsp. |
| Oregano | 3.00 | 20 tbsp. |
| Parsley | 0.37 | 4 cups |

## Condiments & Dressings

| | Calorie Density | Real-Life Conversion |
|---|---|---|
| Barbecue sauce | 1.50 | ¼ cup |
| Blue cheese dressing | 4.67 | 1½ tbsp. |
| Blue cheese dressing, fat-free | 1.00 | 6 tbsp. |
| Cocktail sauce | 0.91 | ¼ cup |
| Honey | 3.05 | 1½ oz. |
| Hot sauce | 0.36 | 25 tbsp. |
| Italian dressing | 3.00 | 2 tbsp. |
| Italian dressing, fat-free | 0.61 | 10 tbsp. |

## Condiments & Dressings (continued)

| | Calorie Density | Real-Life Conversion |
|---|---|---|
| Ketchup | 1.00 | 7 tbsp. |
| Mayo, Primal Kitchen | 6.66 | 1½ tbsp. |
| Mayonnaise, light | 2.33 | 3 tbsp. |
| Mayonnaise, omega light | 3.33 | 2 tbsp. |
| Mayonnaise, real | 6.92 | 1½ tbsp. |
| Mayonnaise, reduced-fat, olive oil | 3.21 | 2 tbsp. |
| Miracle Whip | 2.67 | 2½ tbsp. |
| Miracle Whip, light | 1.31 | 5 tbsp. |
| Mustard | 1.00 | 7 tbsp. |
| Ranch dressing | 4.67 | 1½ tbsp. |
| Ranch dressing, fat-free | 1.47 | 2½ tbsp. |
| Ranch dressing, light | 2.33 | 2½ tbsp. |
| Salsa | 0.36 | 1⅓ cups |
| Soy sauce | 0.67 | 10 tbsp. |
| Teriyaki, ready-to-serve | 0.89 | 6 tbsp. |

## Miscellaneous

| | Calorie Density | Real-Life Conversion |
|---|---|---|
| Anchovy paste | 1.80 | 3⅓ tbsp. |
| Baking flour, enriched | 3.64 | ⅕ cup |
| Baking powder | 1.50 | 33 tsp. |
| Balsamic vinegar | 0.88 | 7 tbsp. |
| Chia flour | 4.89 | 1 tbsp. |
| Chia seed | 3.84 | 2 tbsp. |
| Chocolate chips, carob | 5.33 | 2½ tbsp. |
| Chocolate chips, dark | 4.93 | 1⅓ tbsp. |
| Chocolate chips, semi-sweet | 4.93 | 1⅓ tbsp. |
| Chocolate chips, unsweetened | 3.93 | 110 chips |
| Cocoa powder | 2.22 | ½ cup |
| Coconut milk, canned | 1.83 | ⅕ cup |

## Miscellaneous (continued)

| | Calorie Density | Real-Life Conversion |
|---|---|---|
| Egg Replacer | 3.75 | 8½ tbsp. |
| Ground flax seed | 5.33 | 2 tbsp. |
| Kirkland Chocolate Chip Oatmeal | 3.95 | ½ packet |
| Kirkland Cooked Quinoa | 1.20 | ¼ cup |
| Kirkland Basmati Rice | 3.64 | ⅛ cup |
| Sesame seeds | 5.78 | 2 tbsp. |
| Shirataki Noodles, Miracle Noodle | 0.00 | Unlimited |
| Soy cheese | 2.11 | 1⅓ slice |
| Sugar, white and brown | 3.81 | ⅛ cup |
| Tempeh | 1.96 | ½ serving |
| Tofu, firm | 0.82 | 1½ slices |
| Tofu, light firm | 0.51 | 2 slices |
| Veggie burger patties | 1.27 | ⅔ patty |
| Vinegar | 0.20 | Unlimited |

## Frozen Foods

| | Calorie Density | Real-Life Conversion |
|---|---|---|
| Amy's Enchilada Verde | 1.41 | ¼ container |
| Amy's Indian Vegetable Korma | 1.15 | ⅓ container |
| Amy's Soft Taco Fiesta, Light and Lean | 0.97 | ½ container |
| Amy's Vegetable Pot Pie | 1.98 | ¼ container |
| Lean Cuisine – Angel Hair Pomodoro | 0.89 | ⅓ container |
| Lean Cuisine – Cheddar Bacon Chicken | 0.88 | ½ container |
| Lean Cuisine – Cheese & Tomato Snack Pizza | 1.88 | ½ flatbread |
| Lean Cuisine – Chicken Teriyaki Stir Fry | 1.06 | ½ container |
| Lean Cuisine – Chicken, Spinach & Mushroom Panini | 1.76 | ⅓ container |
| Lean Cuisine – Classic Macaroni & Beef | 1.16 | ⅓ container |
| Lean Cuisine – Lasagna with Meat Sauce | 1.04 | ⅓ container |

# Frozen Foods (continued)

| | Calorie Density | Real-Life Conversion |
|---|---|---|
| Lean Cuisine – Macaroni & Cheese | 1.06 | ⅓ container |
| Lean Cuisine – Pasta Romano with Bacon | 0.92 | ⅓ container |
| Lean Cuisine – Pomegranate Chicken | 0.85 | ½ container |
| Lean Cuisine – Ricotta Cheese and Spinach Ravioli | 1.37 | ⅓ container |
| Lean Cuisine – Roasted Chicken and Garden Vegetables | 0.74 | ½ container |
| Lean Cuisine – Roasted Turkey & Vegetables | 0.88 | ½ container |
| Lean Cuisine – Roasted Turkey Breast | 0.98 | ⅓ container |
| Lean Cuisine – Salisbury Steak with Mac & Cheese | 0.97 | ⅓ container |
| Lean Cuisine – Salmon with Basil | 0.92 | ⅓ container |
| Lean Cuisine – Spaghetti with Meatballs | 0.95 | ⅓ container |
| Lean Cuisine – Steak Portobello | 0.71 | ⅔ container |
| Lean Cuisine – Swedish Meatballs | 1.12 | ⅓ container |
| Lean Cuisine – Sweet & Sour Chicken | 1.06 | ⅓ container |
| Lean Cuisine – Vegetable Eggroll | 1.25 | ⅓ container |

# Beverages

| | Calorie Density | Real-Life Conversion |
|---|---|---|
| Almond milk, sweetened | 0.25 | 14 oz. |
| Almond milk, unsweetened | 0.13 | 3¼ cups |
| Apple juice | 0.46 | 7 oz. |
| Beer, Coors Light | 0.30 | 12 oz. |
| Beer, Michelob Ultra | 0.28 | 12 oz. |
| Beer, Miller Lite | 0.32 | 11 oz. |
| Beer, O'Doul's, nonalcoholic | 0.19 | 18 oz. |
| Coconut milk, sweetened | 0.33 | 10 oz. |
| Coconut milk, unsweetened | 0.19 | 18 oz. |
| Coconut water | 0.19 | 18 oz. |

# Beverages (continued)

| | Calorie Density | Real-Life Conversion |
|---|---|---|
| Coffee, black | 0.00 | Unlimited |
| Coffee, with 2 tbsp. half & half | 0.06 | 7⅓ cups |
| Coffee, with sweetened creamer | 0.10 | 4⅓ cups |
| Espresso | 0.00 | Unlimited |
| Espresso, latte, 1% milk | 0.37 | 9 oz. |
| Espresso, latte, 1% milk, caramel | 0.50 | 7 oz. |
| Espresso, latte, 2% milk | 0.42 | 8 oz. |
| Espresso, latte, 2% milk, caramel | 0.55 | 6 oz. |
| Espresso, latte, half & half | 0.97 | 3 oz. |
| Espresso, latte, half & half, caramel | 1.03 | 3 oz. |
| Espresso, latte, skim milk | 0.29 | 12 oz. |
| Espresso, latte, skim milk, caramel | 0.35 | 10 oz. |
| Espresso, latte, whole milk | 0.49 | 7 oz. |
| Espresso, latte, whole milk, caramel | 0.61 | 5 oz. |
| Ginger ale, Schweppes | 0.35 | 10 oz. |
| Grapefruit juice, light, Ocean Spray | 0.50 | 7 oz. |
| Kirkland Bottled Water | 0.00 | Unlimited |
| Kirkland Coffee Costa Rica | 0.00 | Unlimited |
| Kirkland Coffee Guatemalan Lake Atitlan | 0.00 | Unlimited |
| Kirkland Coffee Panama Geisha | 0.00 | Unlimited |
| Kirkland Coffee Rwanda | 0.00 | Unlimited |
| Kirkland Coffee Sumatra | 0.00 | Unlimited |
| Kirkland Unsweetened Tea | 0.00 | Unlimited |
| Sports drink, Gatorade, lemonade | 0.22 | 16 oz. |
| Tea, unsweetened plain, hot or iced | 0.01 | 44 cups |
| Vegetable juice, V8 100% | 0.22 | 16 oz. |
| Wine, dessert | 1.60 | 2 oz. |
| Wine, red | 0.85 | 4 oz. |
| Wine, white | 0.84 | 4 oz. |

Tiny and Full

# Snacks & Treats

| | Calorie Density | Real-Life Conversion |
|---|---|---|
| Cheetos, crunchy | 5.46 | 14 pieces |
| Cheetos, jumbo cheese puffs | 5.43 | 9 pieces |
| Cheez-its | 4.76 | 17 crackers |
| Doritos, Cool Ranch | 5.36 | 8 chips |
| Granola bar, 25% less sugar | 4.17 | 1 bar |
| Granola bar, chocolate chunk | 3.75 | 1 bar |
| Green and Black's, organic dark 72% chocolate | 3.77 | 5 pieces |
| Green and Black's, organic dark 85% chocolate | 6.25 | 5 pieces |
| Hershey's, milk chocolate | 3.71 | ½ bar |
| Ice cream, soft serve, vanilla | 1.33 | ⅓ cup |
| Kettle chips, lightly salted | 5.28 | 9 chips |
| Nabisco Ritz Crackers, original | 5.03 | 6 crackers |
| Nabisco Ritz Crackers, reduced-fat | 4.67 | 7 crackers |
| Newman's Own, chocolate crème cookies | 4.44 | 1½ cookies |
| Oreo | 4.74 | 2 cookies |
| Oreo, thin crisps | 4.35 | 1 package |
| Pepperidge Farms goldfish crackers | 4.67 | 40 pieces |
| Pirate's Booty | 4.64 | ¾ oz. |
| Popchips, original | 4.30 | 1 small bag |
| Popcorn, air popped | 3.88 | 3 cups |
| Popcorn, kettle corn | 4.15 | 1½ cups |
| Quaker rice cakes, lightly salted | 3.89 | 3 cakes |
| Trail mix | 4.84 | ⅛ cup |
| Wasa Original Crispbread | 4.00 | 1½ slices |
| Wheat Thins | 4.33 | 11 crackers |
| Wheat Thins, reduced fat | 4.48 | 12 crackers |

Tiny and Full™ Foods

# 8 Tiny and Full™ Breakfast Recipes

L et's get shakin'!

I am thrilled to share with you some mouthwatering breakfast recipes to help you Wake Up Vegan™. The breakfasts are divided into two categories.

- Breakfast Boosters: These recipes are my personal favorite and ones I eat regularly. Each of these recipes is designed to give you the extra edge with 10 grams of hunger-fighting pea protein. You can use the Tiny and Full™ pea protein or any other brand of your choosing.

Why pea protein? It is the best solution to the protein powder family. This protein powder holds your appetite the longest. Not only will it keep you fuller for the entire day, it completely staves off hunger for three hours. That means that you can arrive at your next meal feeling ready to eat, but never starving or ravenous. This is the protein powder that will keep you on track to being Tiny, while always being full.

- First and foremost it is a vegan protein, so it goes perfectly with the Tiny and Full philosophy of making delicious quick protein filled vegan breakfasts.

- Secondly it has high bioavailability, which means that it is easy on your digestive tract, absorbed at a high level, and the nutrients are highly available to nourish your body. In other words it doesn't cause any of the problems or issues of the protein powders discussed in the previous paragraphs.

- Third, studies that compare pea protein powders to egg, whey, casein, and soy show that pea protein powders are superior at keeping you full for longer—all day in fact, which is plenty of time to make it from breakfast to lunch without ever getting hungry.

In a study published in the *International Journal of Obesity* in 2008, researchers from The Netherlands and Switzerland who study human biology had 39 overweight men and women, ages 18 to 60 drink a shake made of either whey protein, pea protein, milk protein, or water. After they finished drinking, the participants were asked to rate their hunger every 30 minutes for three hours. Those who had the pea protein reported less desire to eat for the entire three hours than compared to the other proteins. The people in the study who drank the pea protein powder also reported feeling higher levels of fullness.

To sum it up, pea protein powder will provide you with all the benefits of protein—staying full for longer, reducing the drive to eat all day long, eating less calories effortlessly—without all the problems that come with other protein powders. Plus, it's delicious, affordable, and available anywhere protein powders are sold.

- Basic Breakfasts: The second category is regular vegan breakfasts. These do not have pea protein built into the recipe; however, I highly recommend adding it to the meals that you choose. For example, I always add unsweetened pea protein to my oatmeal (see Morning Oats, page 206). Other recipes I recommend adding to: Very Berry Acai Bowl (page 198) and Berry Kiwi Parfait (page 205).

Take note of calorie counts and either adjust portions or reduce snacks throughout the day to make sure you stay within your calorie goal.

## Power Up!

Still hungry? Need an energy boost? If you find yourself a little tired or wanting a bigger breakfast in the morning, add some extra antioxidants and nutrients to your smoothies with my Tiny and Full™ smoothie boosts. I've created two nutrient-rich blends to assist you with your everyday health and wellness. These incredible boosters have tons of antioxidants, vitamins, and important minerals your body needs to maintain a balanced diet.

Pick and choose between my Power Greens boost, which gives you those extra vegetable minerals you are lacking, or my Power Fruits boost, which provides your body with four servings of fruit with just one scoop. Made from more than 30 all-natural ingredients, these smoothie boosts give your body the extra kick it needs and help you feel full with good fiber.

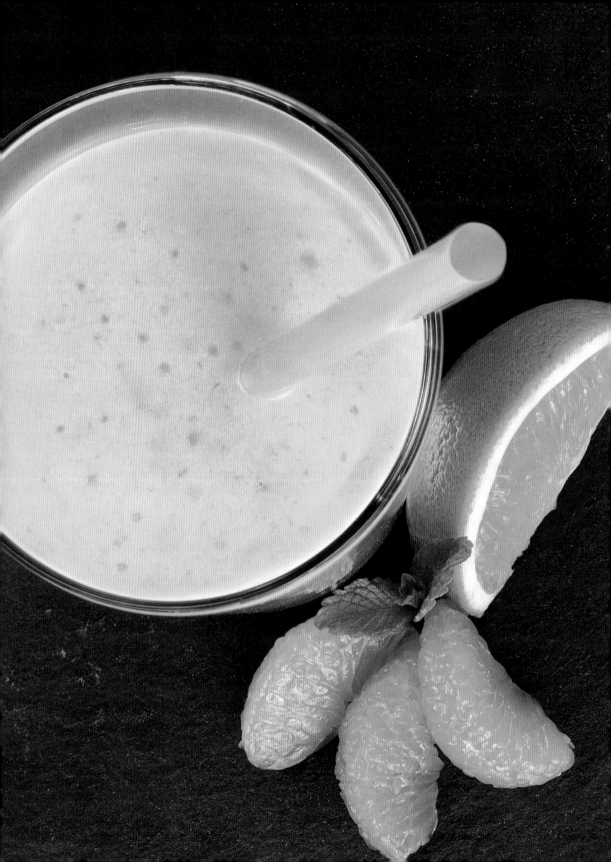

# Breakfast Boosters

## Tropical Mango Blast

**Serves 2**

**243 Calories,** 2.5g Fat, 36.2g Carbs, 25.3g Sugar, 3.4g Fiber, 11.2g Protein

1 cup frozen mango cubes
¾ cup frozen pineapple chunks
1 banana, peeled and cut into large chunks
½–¾ cup unsweetened coconut milk
30 g (about 2 scoops) vanilla pea protein powder

1. Place mango, pineapple, banana, coconut milk, and protein powder in a blender.
2. Blend until completely smooth.
3. Pour into 2 glasses and serve.
4. Sip on!

# Power Greens Smoothie

**Serves 1**

**327 Calories,** 13.6g Fat, 41g Carbs, 24.3g Sugar, 9.1g Fiber, 18.6g Protein

1 large apple, chopped
1 tbsp. almond butter
15 g (about 1 scoop) vanilla pea protein powder
1 cup unsweetened almond milk
4–5 ice cubes
3 cups spinach

1. Place apple, almond butter, protein powder, almond milk, and ice cubes in a blender.
2. Blend until completely smooth.
3. Add spinach in batches, blending a handful at a time until it is all well mixed.
4. Pour into a glass and serve.
5. Enjoy!

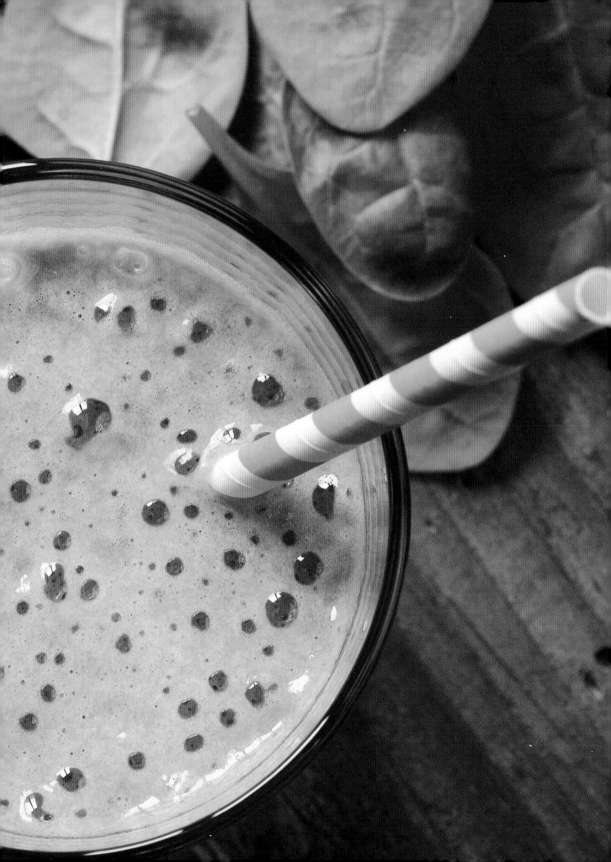

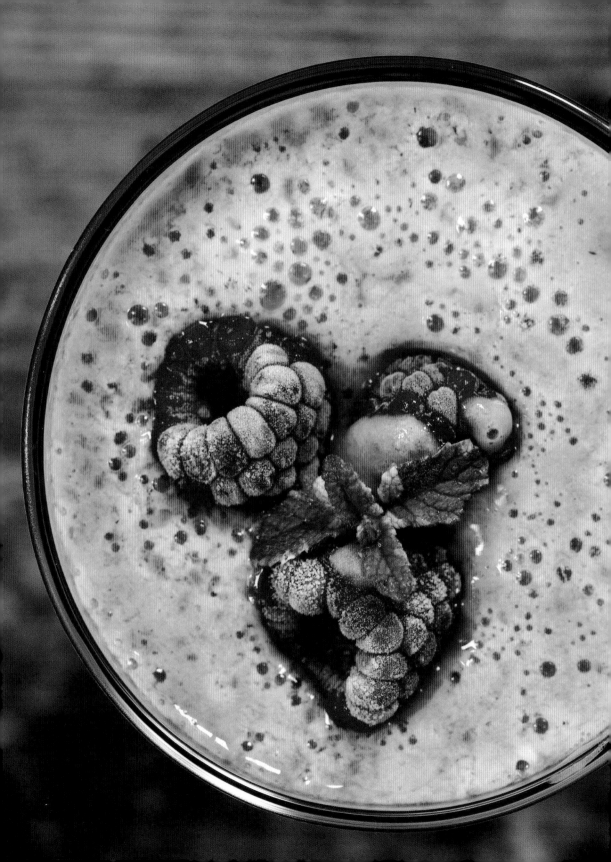

# Minty Detoxer

**Serves 1**

**342 Calories,** 10.5g Fat, 56.3g Carbs, 37.2g Sugar, 13.4g Fiber, 12.9g Protein

1 large fresh orange
½ cup frozen mango cubes
½ cup frozen raspberries
3½ oz. (1 packet) frozen acai puree
15 g (about 1 scoop) unflavored or vanilla pea protein powder
½ cup unsweetened coconut milk
4 fresh mint leaves

For garnish:
3 raspberries
Fresh mint

1. Place all ingredients in a blender.
2. Blend until completely smooth.
3. Pour into a glass and top with garnishes.
4. Serve.
5. Ready. Set. Detox!

# Banana for Berries Bowl

**Serves 2**

**380 Calories,** 14.4g Fat, 78.6g Carbs, 41.4g Sugar, 16.3g Fiber, 15.2g Protein

1 large frozen banana, peeled
¾ cup frozen raspberries
½ cup blueberries
1 tsp. acai berry powder
30 g (about 2 scoops) vanilla pea protein powder
1 cup water
1 tsp. chia seeds

For the toppings:
1 large banana, sliced
¼ cup raspberries
½ cup blueberries
¼ cup blackberries

1. Place all smoothie ingredients except chia seeds in a blender and puree until smooth.
2. Stir in chia seeds.
3. Allow mixture to sit for about 5 minutes. This will allow the chia seeds to absorb some of the water and make the smoothie thicker.
4. Blend one more time, and then pour it into two bowls.
5. Top with fruit garnishes and serve. Dig in!

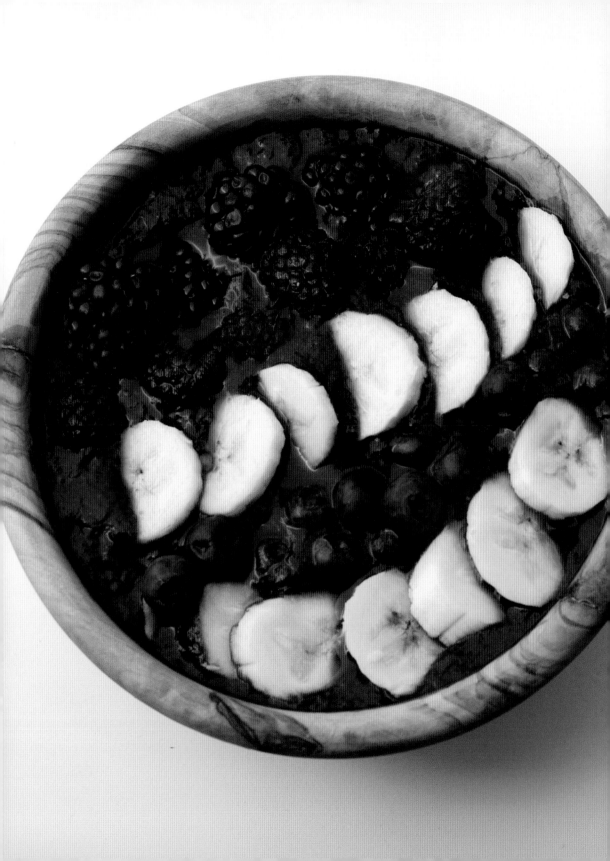

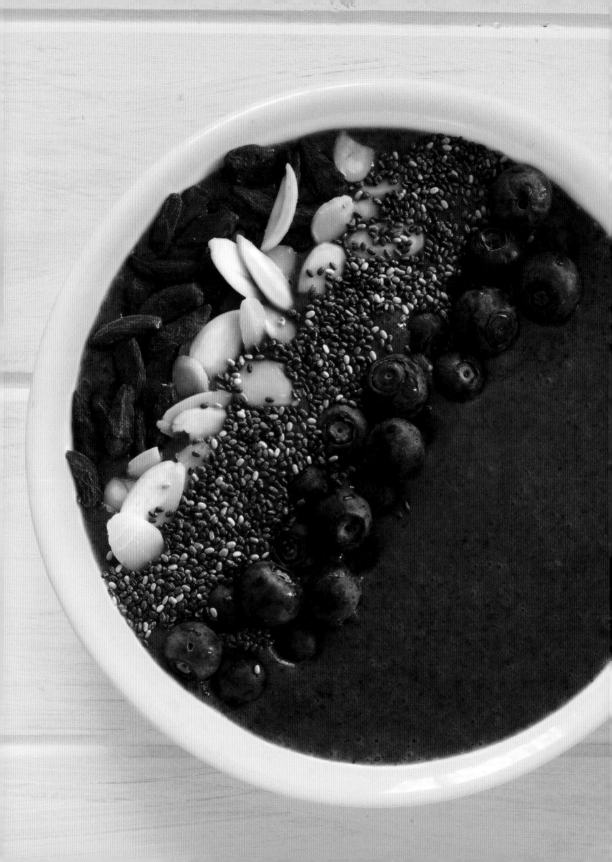

# Berry Blaster Bowl

**Serves 2**

**273 Calories,** 6.6g Fat, 45.8g Carbs, 27.1g Sugar, 16.2g Fiber, 24.6g Protein

1 cup baby spinach
1 tbsp. chia seeds
1½ cups unsweetened almond milk
1½ cups frozen mixed berries
15 g (about 1 scoop) unsweetened or vanilla pea protein powder
½ frozen banana, peeled
1 tsp. light agave nectar

For the toppings:
¼ cup blueberries
1 tsp. chia seeds
2 tbsp. slivered almonds
1 tbsp. goji berries

1. Place spinach, chia seeds, and almond milk in a blender and mix until smooth.
2. Add frozen mixed berries, protein powder, banana, and agave.
3. Blend, making sure to scrape down the sides of the blender every so often, until smooth.
4. Pour into a bowl and garnish with toppings.
5. Serve immediately. Enjoy!

# Dragon Fruit Booster Bowl

**Serves 2**

**404 Calories,** 3.4g Fat, 59.2g Carbs, 58.9g Sugar, 11.5g Fiber, 19.6g Protein

1 cup frozen mango cubes
1 cup frozen pineapple chunks
3½ oz. (1 packet) frozen pitaya (dragon fruit) puree
1 cup baby spinach
½ kiwi, peeled
½ cup unsweetened almond milk
30 g (about 2 scoops) unflavored or vanilla pea protein powder

For the toppings:
½ banana, sliced
14 blueberries
10 blackberries
2 tsp. chia seeds
2 tbsp. pumpkin seeds
2 tbsp. almonds

1. Place all smoothie ingredients in a blender and blend until smooth.
2. Pour into a serving bowl and top with the fresh fruits, seeds, and nuts, as desired.
3. Serve immediately. Dig in!

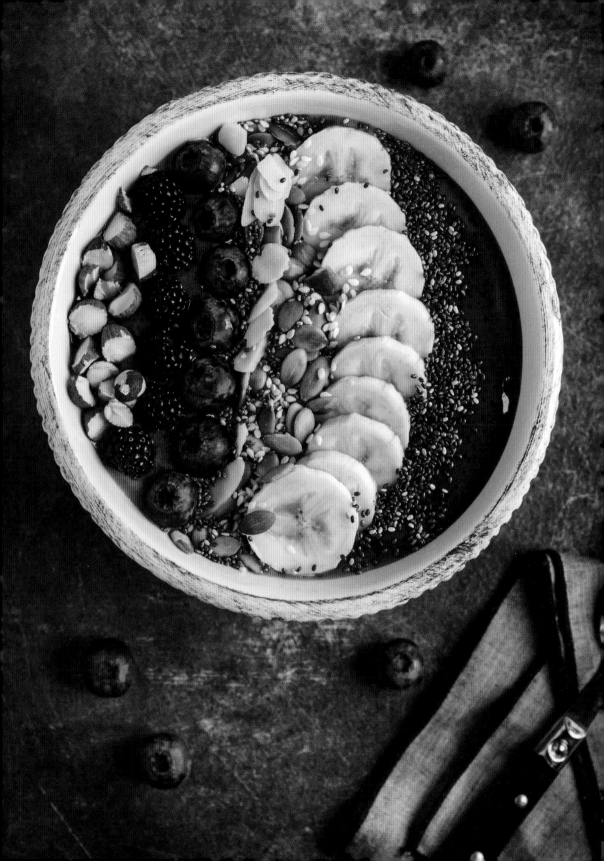

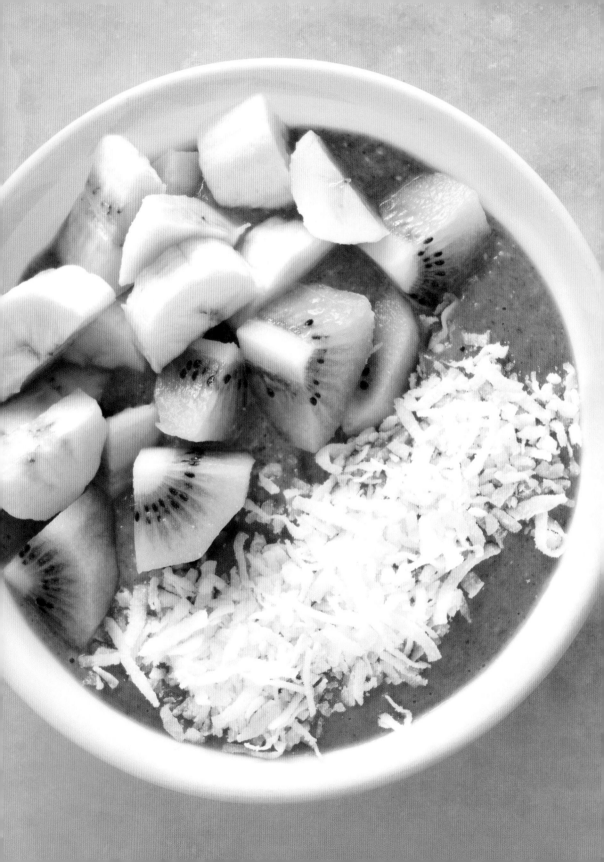

# Sweet Greens Smoothie Bowl

**Serves 1**

**341 Calories,** 14.1g Fat, 43.5g Carbs, 22.4g Sugar, 78.3g Fiber, 15.6g Protein

1 cup unsweetened almond milk
½ cup frozen mango cubes
15 g (about 1 scoop) vanilla pea protein powder
½ avocado
1 cup kale
1 cup spinach
2 ice cubes
¼ cup cold water, more as needed

For the toppings:
¼ cup sliced banana
¼ cup sliced kiwi
2 tbsp. unsweetened coconut flakes

1. Place almond milk, mango, protein powder, avocado, kale, spinach, and ice cubes in a blender and blend until smooth.

2. Add cold water as needed, to desired thickness, and blend again.

3. Pour into a serving bowl and top with fruit and coconut flakes, as desired.

4. Serve immediately. Dig in!

# Blueberry Kickstarter

**Serves 1**

**206 Calories,** 1.4g Fat, 40.1g Carbs, 27.9g Sugar, 4.6g Fiber, 12g Protein

1 cup chopped green melon
½ cup blueberries
1 medium banana, peeled
¼ cup water
15 g (about 1 scoop) vanilla pea protein powder
Ice, to desired thickness

1. Place all ingredients in a blender.
2. Blend until completely smooth.
3. Pour into a glass and serve.
4. Sit back, relax, and sip.

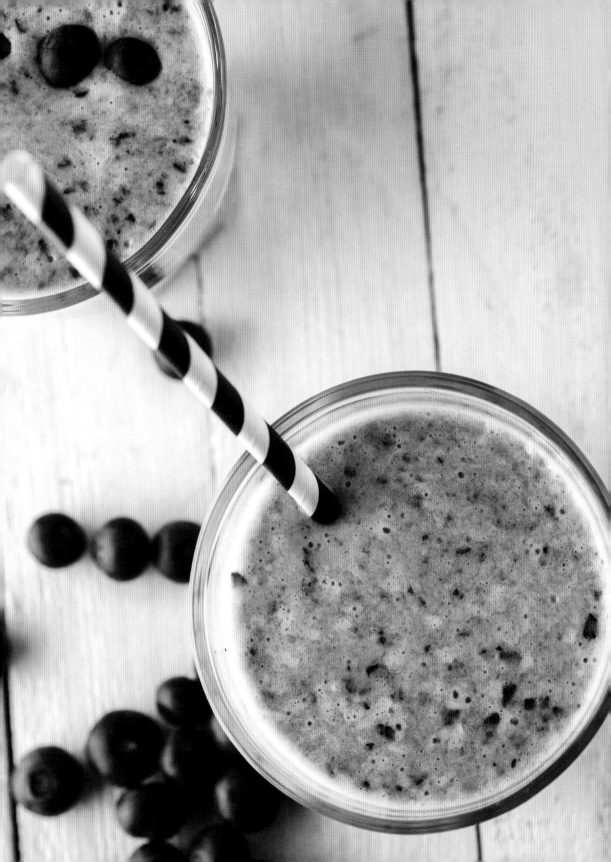

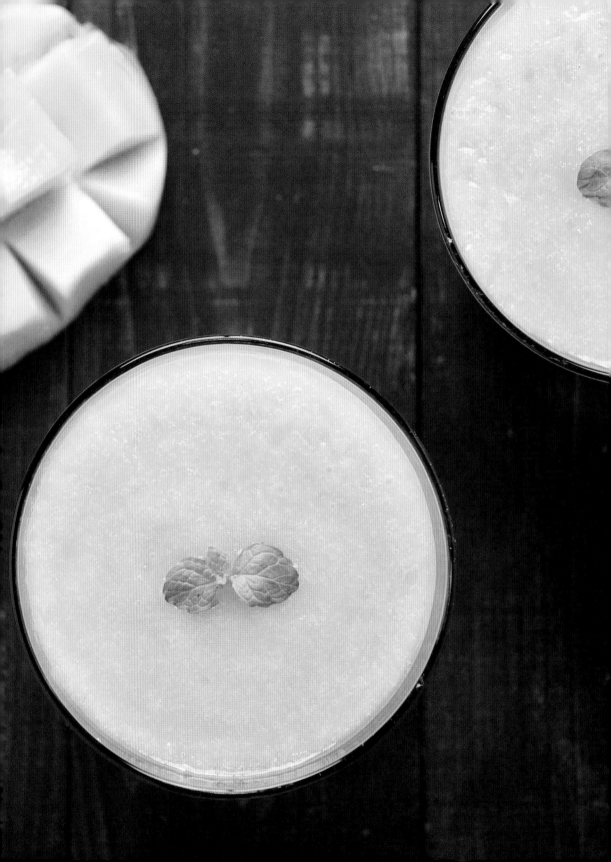

# Sunrise Smoothie

**Serves 1**

**199 Calories,** 1.7g Fat, 54.4g Carbs, 35.1g Sugar, 5.1g Fiber, 13g Protein

½ cup freshly squeezed orange juice
½ cup tangerine slices
1 medium banana, peeled
15 g (about 1 scoop) vanilla pea protein powder
Ice, to desired thickness

1. Place all ingredients in a blender.
2. Blend until completely smooth.
3. Pour into a glass and serve. Cheers!

# Cocoa Banana Bowl

**Serves 4**

**456 Calories,** 20.6g Fat, 57.1g Carbs, 26.3g Sugar, 11.6g Fiber, 20.3g Protein

1 cup unsweetened coconut milk

4 bananas (2 of them frozen), peeled

2 tbsp. peanut butter

½ cup unsweetened cocoa powder

60 g (about 4 scoops) chocolate pea protein powder

For the toppings:

1 banana, sliced

¼ cup dark chocolate shavings

15 pieces unsweetened coconut slices

¼ cup almonds

1. Place all smoothie ingredients in a blender.
2. Blend until completely smooth.
3. Pour into a bowl and garnish with toppings, as desired.
4. Serve immediately. Dig in!

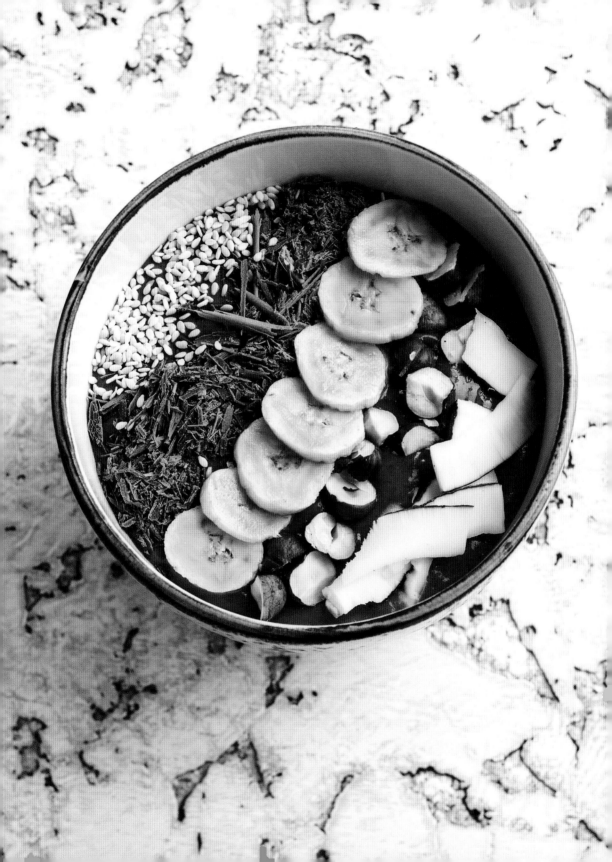

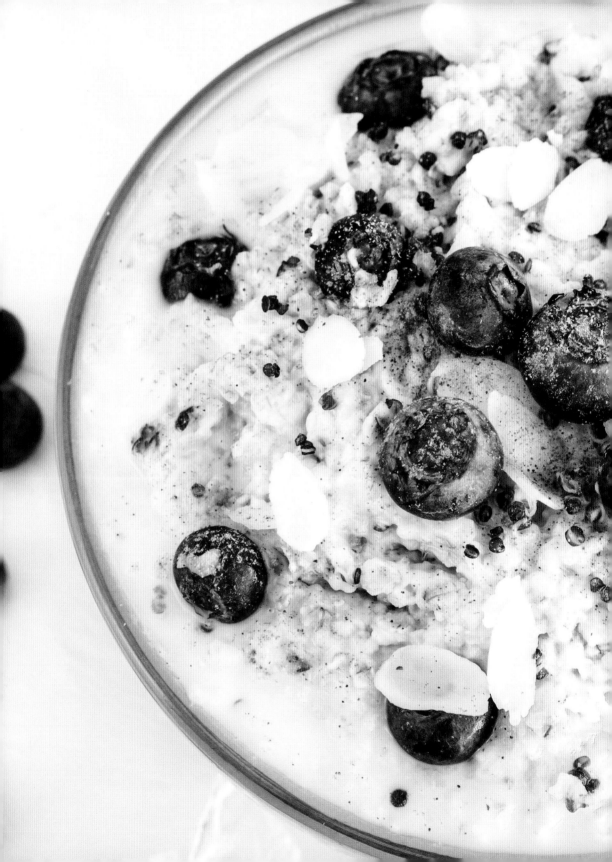

# Basic Breakfasts

## Sunshine Cinnamon Nut Quinoa

**Serves 4**

**274 Calories,** 8g Fat, 44.2g Carbs, 11.2g Sugar, 6.2g Fiber, 8.7g Protein

1 cup unsweetened almond milk
1 cup water
1 cup quinoa, rinsed
⅓ cup slivered almonds, toasted
½ tsp. ground cinnamon
2 cups fresh blueberries
4 tsp. agave nectar

1.  Combine almond milk, water, and quinoa in a medium saucepan.
2.  Bring to a boil over high heat.
3.  Reduce heat to medium-low, cover, and simmer for 15 minutes, or until most of the liquid is absorbed.
4.  Turn off heat; let stand, covered, for 5 minutes.
5.  While quinoa cooks, preheat toaster to 350°F.
6.  Spread almonds on a small baking sheet and toast for 4–6 minutes, or toast in a dry skillet over medium heat for 2–3 minutes.
7.  Stir cinnamon into the quinoa.
8.  Divide quinoa among four bowls and top with almonds and blueberries.
9.  Drizzle 1 tsp. agave nectar over each serving. You can add more almond milk, if desired.
10. *Bon appetit*!

# Good Morning Chia Seed Pudding

**Serves 4**

**216 Calories,** 10.9g Fat, 26.6g Carbs, 10.9g Sugar, 12.7g Fiber, 5.7g Protein

3 cups unsweetened almond milk
½ cup chia seeds
1 tbsp. pure maple syrup, or to taste
1 cup blueberries
¾ cup chopped mango

For the toppings:
12 blueberries

1. In a large bowl, whisk together almond milk, chia seeds, and maple syrup.
2. Let sit for 5–10 minutes. Whisk again.
3. Cover and place in the fridge for 2½–3 hours. You can also let it chill overnight. Stir mixture occasionally.
4. Remove from fridge and stir. Mix in blueberries and chopped mango.
5. Divide among four bowls and top with additional blueberries.
6. Enjoy!

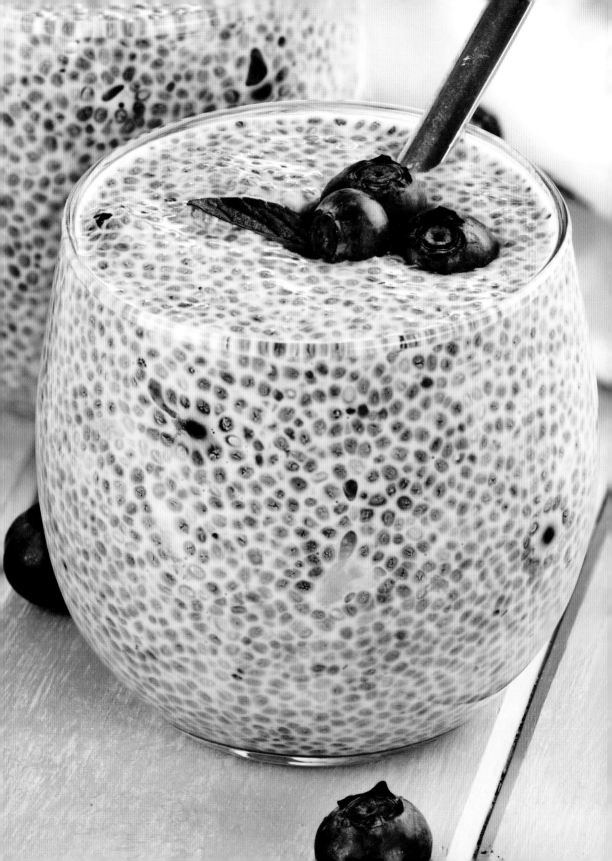

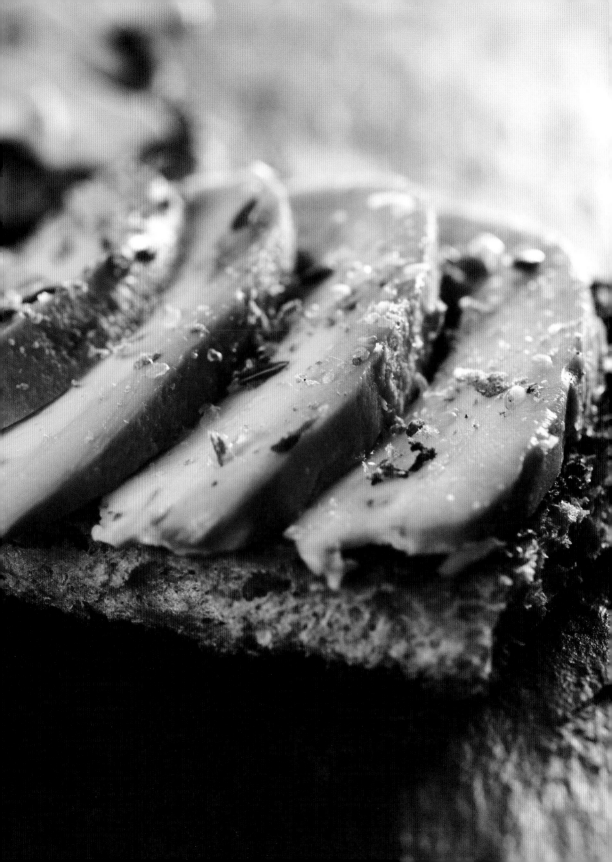

# Hummus Avocado Toast

**Serves 1**

**363 Calories,** 13.4g Fat, 10.2g Carbs, 0.5g Sugar, 6.6g Fiber, 3.7g Protein

2 slices vegan whole-wheat bread
2 tbsp. hummus
8 slices avocado
Himalayan pink salt and pepper, to taste

1. Toast bread to desired doneness.
2. Spread each slice with 1 tbsp. hummus.
3. Top with avocado slices.
4. Sprinkle with salt and pepper.
5. Get eating!

# Wake-Up French Toast

**Serves 4**

**395 Calories,** 1.9g Fat, 86.6g Carbs, 43.3g Sugar, 4.5g Fiber, 9.8g Protein

1 ripe banana, peeled
1 cup unsweetened almond milk
½ tsp. ground cinnamon
¼ tsp. vanilla extract
8 slices vegan whole-wheat bread
½ cup maple syrup
1 cup halved grapes
4 strawberries, sliced
1 passion fruit, sliced
1 orange, peeled and sliced
1 kiwi, sliced

1. In a small bowl, use a fork to mash banana. Add almond milk, cinnamon, and vanilla and mix together well.

2. Heat a pan over medium heat. Spray with cooking spray.

3. Dip one slice of bread at a time in the banana-almond milk mixture, making sure to wet both sides.

4. Place bread in hot pan. Cook on each side for 4 minutes, or until golden brown.

5. Serve two pieces per person. Lightly drizzle each with 2 tbsp. maple syrup and top with one-fourth of the fresh fruit.

6. Enjoy!

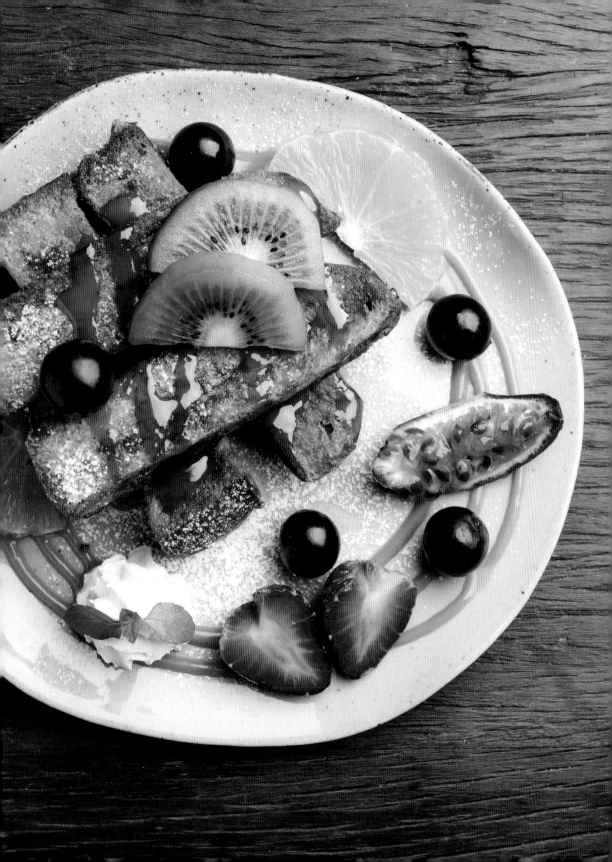

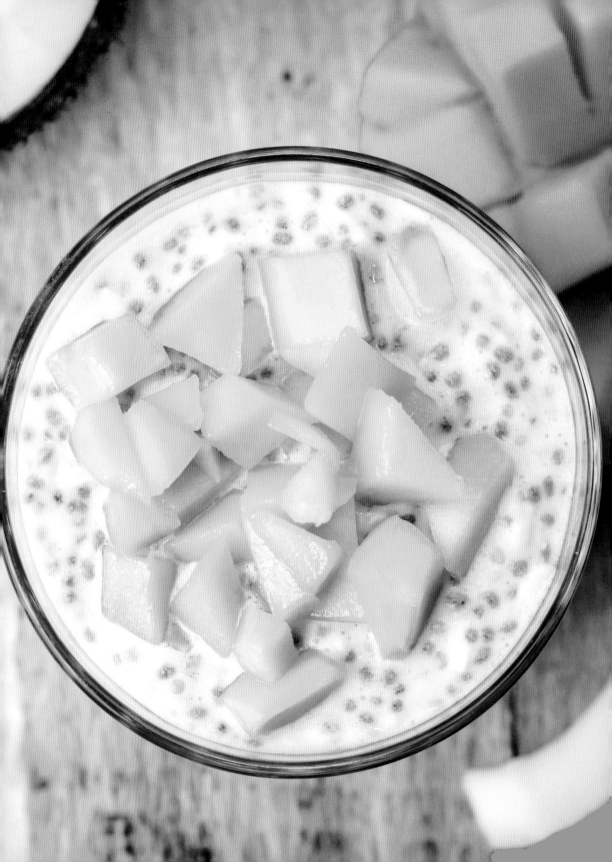

# Coconut Chia Pudding

**Serves 1**

**358 Calories,** 20.6g Fat, 44.3g Carbs, 15.7g Sugar, 22.1g Fiber, 13.2g Protein

¼ cup chia seeds
1 cup unsweetened coconut milk
½ tbsp. agave nectar
¼ cup diced mango

1. In a small bowl, mix together chia seeds, coconut milk, and agave nectar.
2. Cover and refrigerate overnight.
3. Remove from fridge, making sure the pudding looks thick and the chia seeds have gelled.
4. Top with diced mango and serve immediately.
5. Dig in!

# Very Berry Acai Bowl

**Serves 2**

**303 Calories,** 8.1g Fat, 50.3g Carbs, 23.8g Sugar, 9.8g Fiber, 5.6g Protein

2 frozen bananas, sliced
2 cups (10½ oz.) frozen strawberries
4 tbsp. acai powder
1 cup unsweetened almond milk, plus more as needed
½ tbsp. agave nectar

For the toppings:
½ banana, sliced
¼ cup sliced strawberries
¼ cup raspberries
2 tbsp. blueberries

1. Place frozen banana slices, frozen strawberries, acai powder, almond milk, and agave nectar into a blender.

2. Blend until creamy and smooth, adding extra almond milk as needed. (It should be thicker than a smoothie.)

3. Spoon mixture into bowls and top with sliced bananas, strawberries, raspberries, and blueberries.

4. Enjoy!

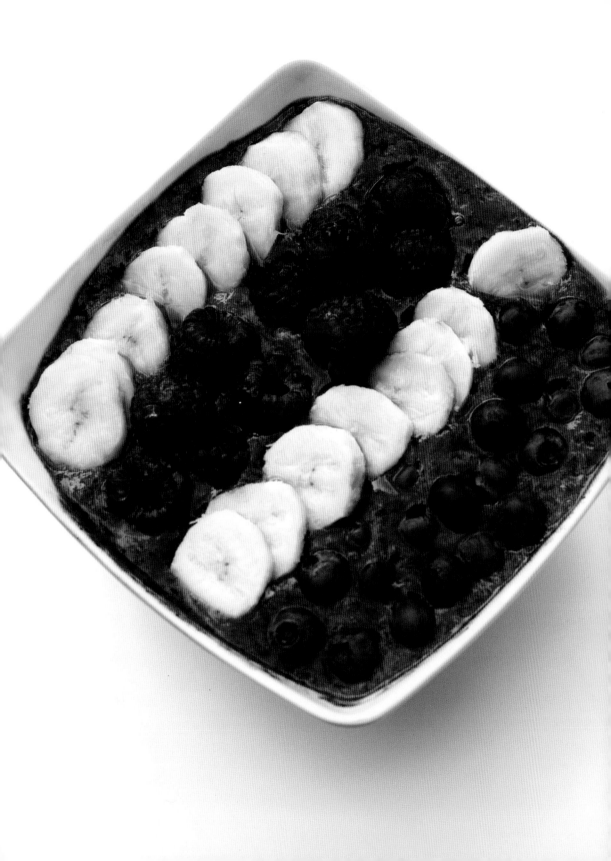

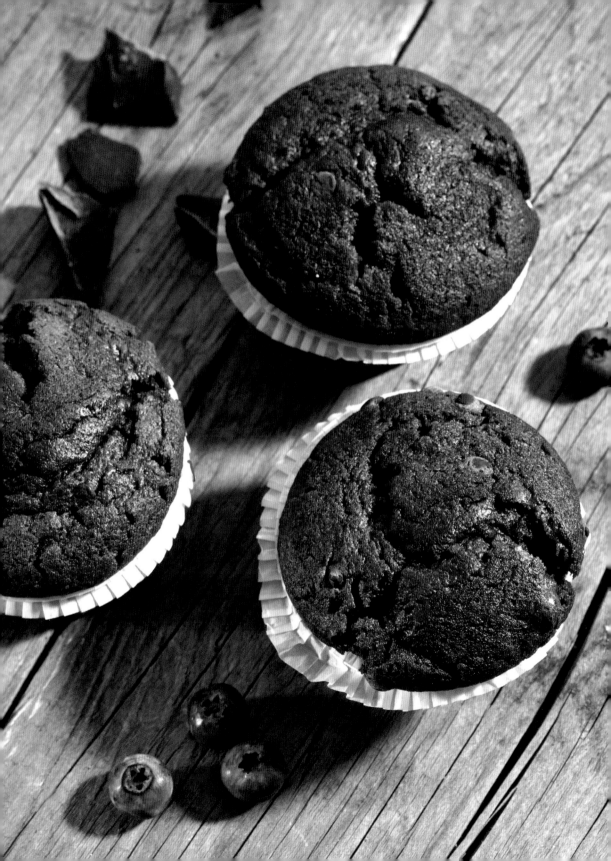

# Chocolate Blueberry Muffins

**Makes 12**

**[Per Muffin] 64 Calories,** 0.9g Fat, 14.9g Carbs, 3.4g Sugar, 1.9g Fiber, 2g Protein

1½ cups all-purpose flour
½ cup unsweetened cocoa powder
4 tsp. raw sugar
2 tsp. baking powder
1½ tsp. egg replacer
½ tsp. salt
1¼ cups unsweetened coconut milk
¼ cup applesauce
½ cup frozen blueberries

1. Preheat oven to 400°F.
2. Spray a 12-cup muffin tin with nonstick cooking spray.
3. In a large bowl, combine flour, cocoa powder, sugar, baking powder, egg replacer, and salt.
4. In a small bowl, mix coconut milk and applesauce.
5. Add wet ingredients to dry ingredients and stir to combine.
6. Fold in blueberries.
7. Using a ¼-cup measure, scoop batter into muffin tins about two-thirds full.
8. Bake for 20–25 minutes, or until toothpick inserted into center comes out clean.
9. Cool for 5 minutes in the tin, and then remove and let cool on a rack.
10. Enjoy!

# Antioxidant Fruit Salad

**Serves 4**

**275 Calories,** 1.3g Fat, 60.3g Carbs, 51.3g Sugar, 10.6g Fiber, 4.3g Protein

Juice of ½ lemon
1 tbsp. agave nectar
4 cups trimmed, halved strawberries
1½ cups blueberries
4 oranges, peeled and chopped
4 kiwis, sliced
3 cups halved red grapes

1. In a small bowl, mix together lemon juice and agave nectar.
2. In a large bowl, mix together fruit.
3. Pour sweetened lemon juice over fruit mixture and toss to coat.
4. Serve immediately or chill until ready.
5. Enjoy!

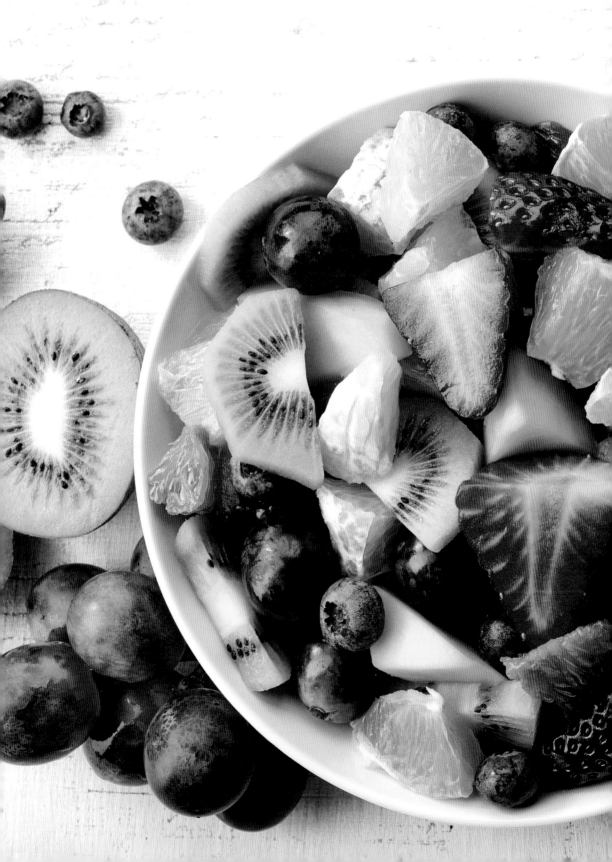

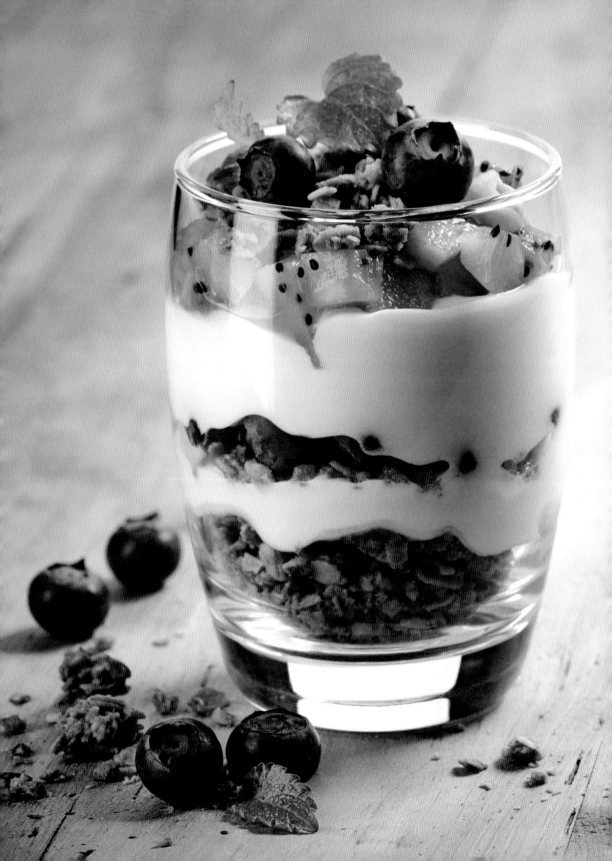

# Berry Kiwi Parfait

**Serves 1**

**339 Calories,** 12.6g Fat, 56.2 Carbs, 30.9g Sugar, 10.3g Fiber, 6.2g Protein

½ cup unsweetened coconut yogurt
Fresh lemon juice and lemon zest, to taste
¼ cup granola
½ cup blueberries
½ cup chopped kiwi
Fresh mint, for garnish (optional)

1. In a small bowl, mix together coconut yogurt, lemon juice, and lemon zest.
2. Put half of the granola in bottom of a serving glass.
3. Layer yogurt, fruit, and remaining granola.
4. Top with a mint leaf, if desired.
5. Enjoy!

# Morning Oats

**Serves 1**

**363 Calories,** 14.7g Fat, 50.1g Carbs, 12.8g Sugar, 19.5g Fiber, 9.2g Protein

½ cup rolled oats
½ cup unsweetened almond milk
2 tbsp. chopped pecans
½ tbsp. pure maple syrup
½ tsp. ground cinnamon
¼ banana, sliced
3 strawberries, sliced

1. In a bowl, mix together oats and almond milk.
2. Cover and refrigerate overnight.
3. The next day, in a small saucepan, heat oat mixture until hot.
4. Add more almond milk, if desired.
5. Pour oats into a bowl and mix with pecans, syrup, and cinnamon.
6. Top with sliced fruit and serve immediately.
7. Dig in!

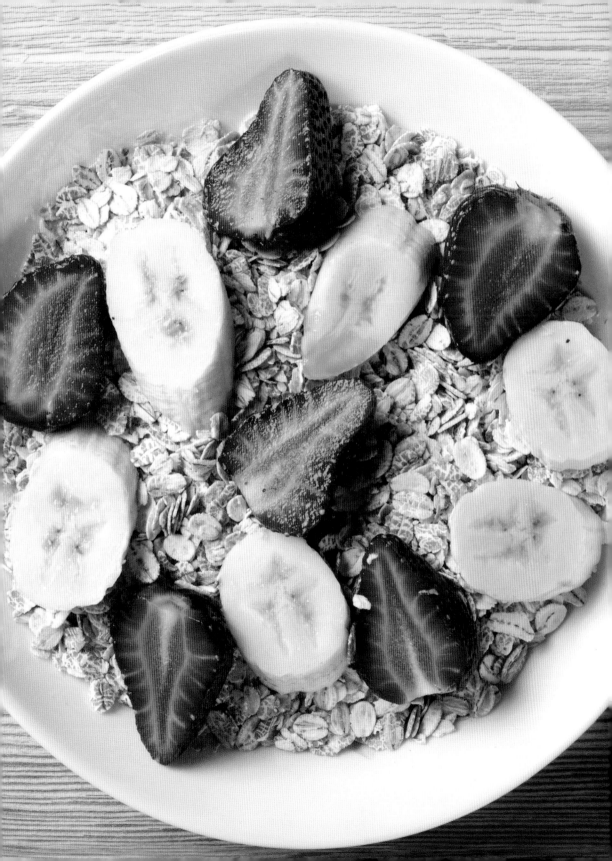

# 9 Tiny and Full™ Entrée Recipes

Let's get cookin'!

And now, I am pleased to introduce you to 20 lunch and dinner options that bring in animal-based foods. The meals are meant to be low in caloric density and are heavily plant focused, but bring a balance of animal-based foods and protein.

Take note of calorie counts and either adjust portions or reduce snacks throughout the day to make sure you stay within your calorie goal.

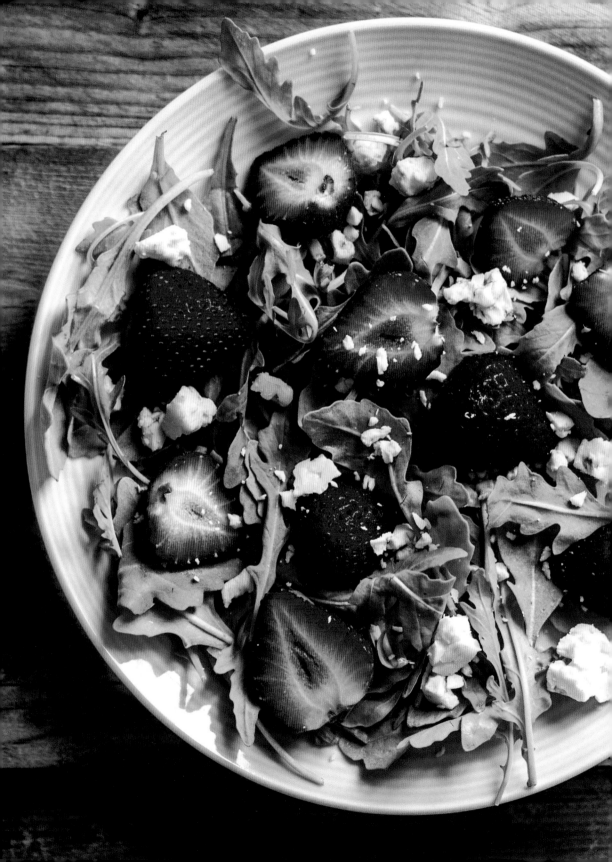

# Strawberry Feta Summer Salad

**Serves 4**

**166 Calories,** 10.8g Fat, 10.6g Carbs, 6.8g Sugar, 3.2g Fiber, 9g Protein

12 cups arugula
1 cup herb sprigs, such as chives, chervil, or mint
3 tbsp. sherry vinaigrette
1 cup crumbled feta cheese
1 cup sliced small strawberries

1. In a large bowl, place greens and herbs and toss to combine.
2. Add vinaigrette and gently toss to coat.
3. Top with feta cheese and strawberries.
4. Divide among four plates and serve.
5. Enjoy!

# Organic Chicken Caesar Salad

**Serves 4**

**310 Calories,** 18.3g Fat, 11g Carbs, 1.9g Sugar, 2.5g Fiber, 25.2g Protein

For the dressing:
½ small clove garlic
⅛ tsp. salt
2 tbsp. lemon juice
1 tbsp. mayonnaise
1 tsp. Dijon mustard
¾ tsp. anchovy paste, or to taste (optional)
¼ tsp. freshly ground pepper
4 tsp. extra virgin olive oil
2 tbsp. grated Asiago cheese

For the salad:
12 oz. boneless, skinless chicken
    breasts, trimmed of fat
1 tsp. extra virgin olive oil
¼ tsp. salt, or to taste
Freshly ground pepper, to taste
8 cups torn romaine lettuce
1 cup croutons
½ cup grated Parmesan cheese

For the dressing:

1. In a medium bowl, place garlic and salt and mash with the back of a spoon to form a paste.
2. Add lemon juice, mayonnaise, mustard, anchovy paste (if desired), and pepper. Whisk together.
3. Slowly drizzle in oil, whisking constantly.
4. Add cheese and whisk to combine.

For the salad:

5. Prepare a grill or preheat broiler.
6. Rub chicken with oil and season with salt and pepper.
7. Grill or broil chicken until browned and no longer pink, 3–4 minutes per side.
8. Combine lettuce and croutons in a large bowl.
9. Toss with the dressing and divide among four plates.
10. Slice chicken and fan over salad.
11. Top with Parmesan.
12. Serve immediately.
13. Dig in!

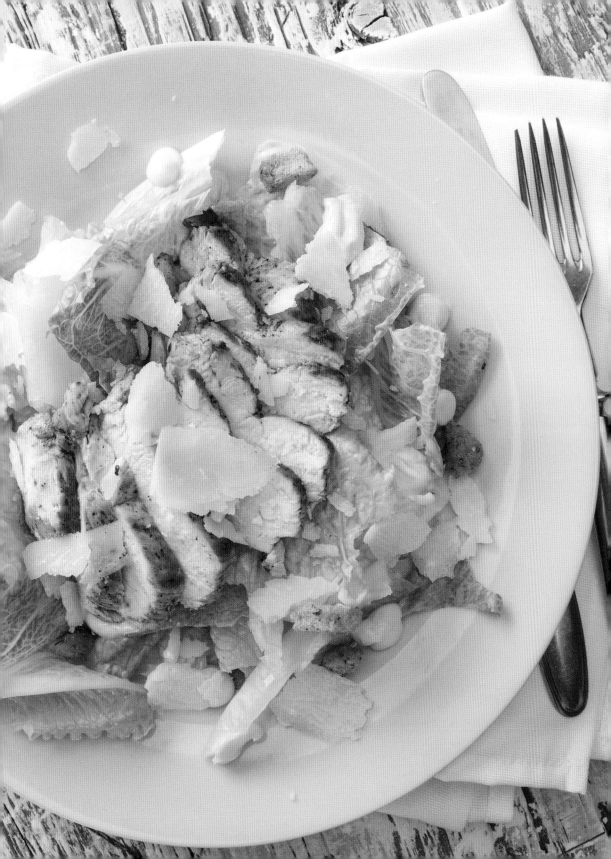

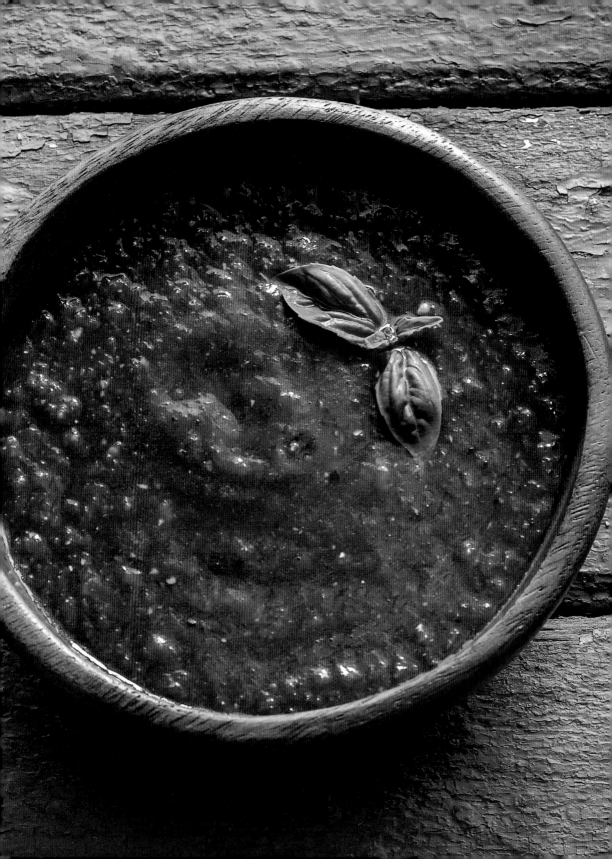

# Tomato Gazpacho Fresca

**Serves 2**

**146 Calories,** 2.9g Fat, 26g Carbs, 13.2g Sugar, 3.6g Fiber, 11g Protein

1 large clove garlic, pressed and chopped

2 shallots, finely sliced

1 tsp. olive oil

1 tsp. brown sugar

2 tbsp. balsamic vinegar, divided

4 tomatoes, quartered

1 roasted red pepper, blotted of oil and moisture

4 ice cubes

⅔ cup plain Greek yogurt

½ tsp. salt

½ tsp. freshly ground black pepper

8 basil leaves, chopped

1. In a nonstick pan over medium heat, sauté garlic and shallots in olive oil until fragrant, approximately 2 minutes.

2. Mix in brown sugar and 1 tbsp. balsamic vinegar.

3. Continue to heat until shallots have softened and vinegar has thickened, approximately 2 minutes.

4. Remove from heat and add to blender.

5. Add tomatoes, remaining 1 tbsp. vinegar, roasted red pepper, ice, yogurt, salt, and pepper and blend until smooth.

6. Transfer to a bowl and place in refrigerator to chill for a minimum of 20 minutes.

7. Divide between two bowls, top with basil, and serve.

8. *Buen provecho*!

# Sweet Arugula Pear Salad

**Serves 4**

**210 Calories,** 12g Fat, 23.3g Carbs, 14.1g Sugar, 4.7g Fiber, 5.9g Protein

6 cups arugula
½ cup crumbled blue cheese
⅓ cup pine nuts
2 large pears, cored and sliced
Balsamic vinegar
Salt and pepper, to taste

1. In a large bowl, combine arugula, blue cheese, and pine nuts.
2. Toss to mix.
3. Divide salad mixture among four plates and top with slices of pear.
4. Lightly drizzle with balsamic vinegar and season with salt and pepper.
5. Enjoy!

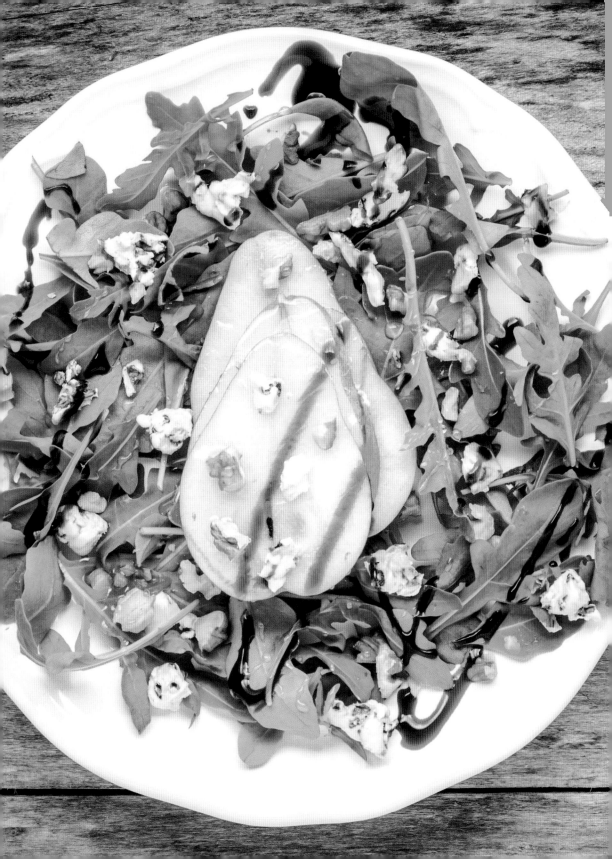

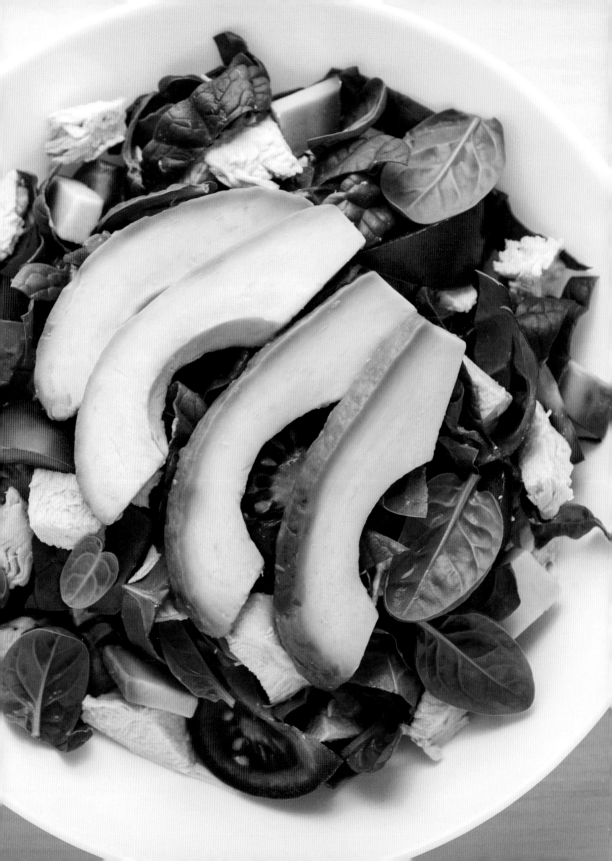

# Turkocado Salad

**Serves 4**

**238 Calories,** 13.5g Fat, 7.3g Carbs, 1g Sugar, 4.9g Fiber, 23.2g Protein

12 oz. turkey breast cutlets
3 tsp. olive oil, divided
¼ tsp. salt, divided
2 tbsp. apple cider vinegar
1 tsp. Dijon mustard
1 tbsp. water
8 cups baby spinach leaves
4 cherry tomatoes, halved
1 oz. goat cheese, crumbled
1 ripe avocado, peeled, pitted, and sliced
Black pepper, to taste

1. Preheat nonstick pan over medium high for approximately 2 minutes.
2. Brush turkey with 1 tsp. of oil and sprinkle with ⅛ tsp. of the salt.
3. Sauté for 4 minutes, flip, and continue cooking until no longer pink and juices run clear.
4. Remove from pan and cut into chunks.
5. In a small bowl, mix together vinegar, mustard, water, remaining 2 tsp. oil, and remaining ⅛ tsp. salt.
6. In a large bowl, toss together spinach, tomatoes, turkey, and cheese with 2 tbsp. of the dressing.
7. Divide among four plates and drizzle with remaining dressing.
8. Top with avocado slices and season with black pepper.
9. Dig in!

# Chicken Veggie Sandwich

**Serves 1**

**398 Calories,** 3.9g Fat, 45g Carbs, 11.1g Sugar, 7g Fiber, 46.3g Protein

2 slices bread
2 tbsp. plain hummus
3 oz. cooked chicken breast, chopped
2 slices low-fat Swiss cheese
4 slices tomato
Basil leaves

1. Toast bread, if desired.
2. Spread hummus on each slice of bread.
3. Add chicken, cheese, tomatoes, and basil.
4. Enjoy.

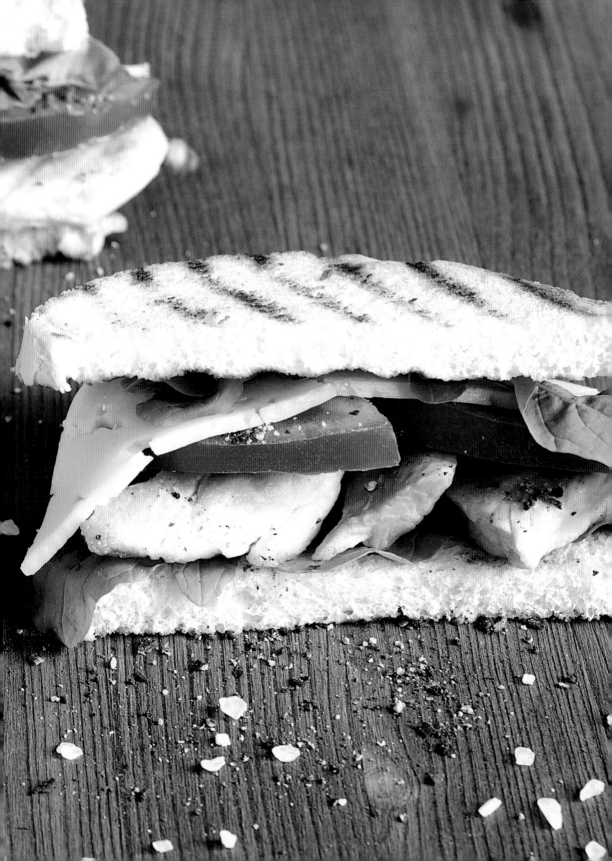

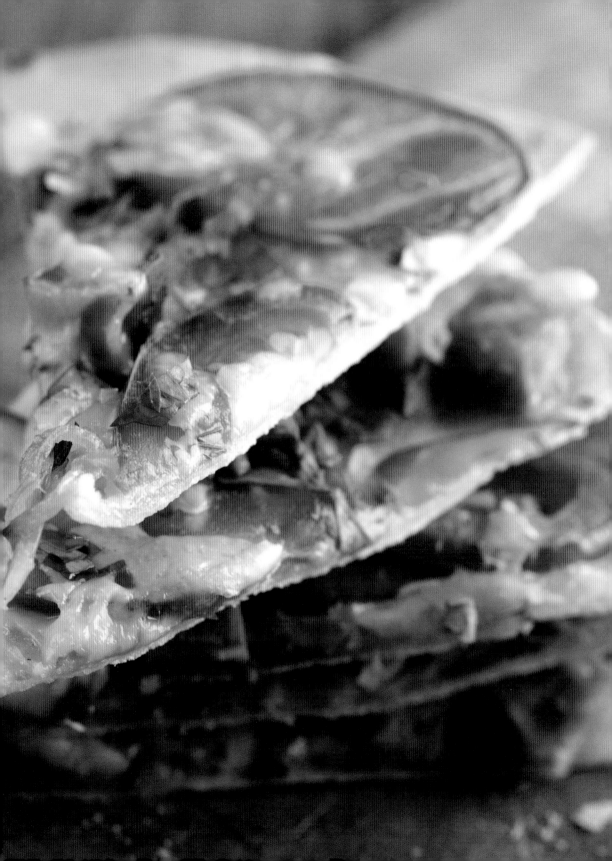

# Tortilla Bacon Mozzarella Pizza

**Serves 1**

**357 Calories,** 6.6g Fat, 30.5g Carbs, 4.7g Sugar, 3.9g Fiber, 29.5g Protein

2 slices bacon, chopped

1 (10-inch) flour tortilla

½ cup shredded mozzarella cheese

1 tbsp. grated Parmesan cheese

½ tomato, thinly sliced

1 clove garlic, minced

4 fresh basil leaved, thinly sliced

1. Preheat oven to 450°F.
2. In a skillet over medium heat, fry bacon until cooked through.
3. Drain on paper towels.
4. Place tortilla on baking sheet.
5. Top with cheeses, tomato slices, and cooked bacon and sprinkle with garlic.
6. Bake for 8–10 minutes, or until tortilla is crisp and cheese is melted.
7. Sprinkle with basil.
8. Slice and serve.
9. Enjoy.

# Sunshine Summer Salad

**Serves 2**

**289 Calories,** 21.5g Fat, 5.5g Carbs, 0.3g Sugar, 0.4g Fiber, 21.8g Protein

8 skewers
8 melon balls
8 mozzarella balls
8 thin slices prosciutto
8 pitted green olives
1 tsp. balsamic vinegar
Basil leaves, torn

1. If using wooden skewers, soak in water for 30 minutes so food won't stick.
2. On each skewer, layer a melon ball, mozzarella ball, and folded-up slice of prosciutto.
3. Place skewers on a plate.
4. Add olives around and lightly drizzle with balsamic vinegar.
5. Garnish with basil leaves.
6. *Buon appetito*!

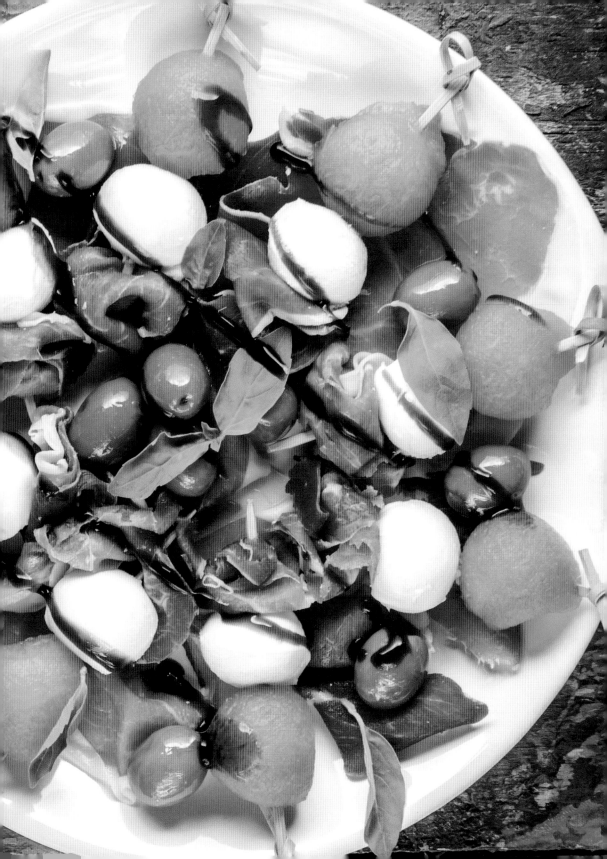

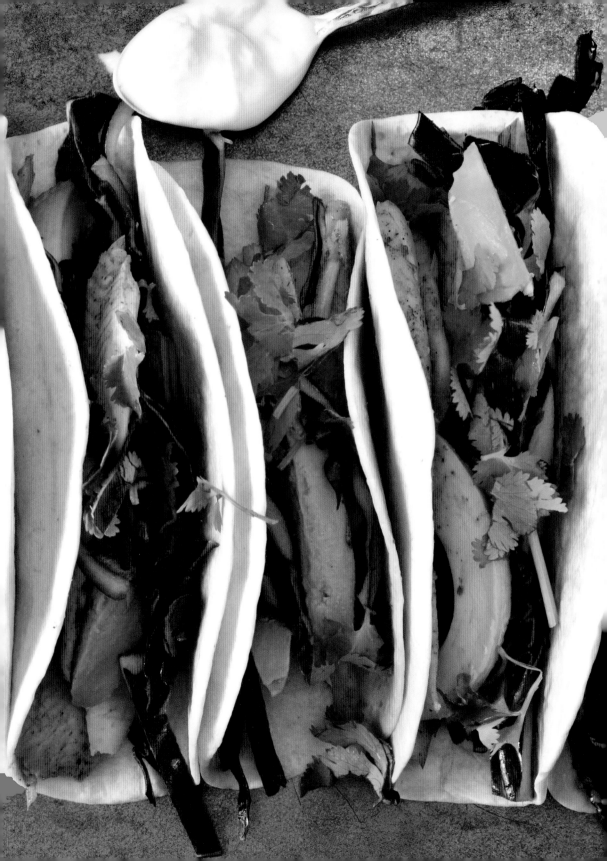

# California Fish Tacos

**Serves 4**

**251 Calories,** 9.8g Fat, 23.3g Carbs, 4.3g Sugar, 4.6g Fiber, 20.4g Protein

1 tbsp. olive oil, plus more for grill
4 (3-oz.) tilapia, halibut, or black bass fillets
1 tsp. ground coriander
¾ tsp. kosher salt, divided
½ tsp. black pepper, divided
6 radishes, sliced
1 cucumber, halved and sliced
2 tbsp. fresh lime juice, plus lime wedges for serving
8 corn tortillas
1 cup fresh cilantro leaves
½ cup chopped purple cabbage
½ avocado, sliced

1. Heat grill to high and oil grill.
2. Season fish fillets with coriander, ½ tsp. of salt, and ¼ tsp. of pepper.
3. Grill until cooked through, 1–2 minutes per side.
4. Break into small to medium-size pieces.
5. In a medium bowl, toss together radishes and cucumber with lime juice, remaining 1 tbsp. oil, remaining ¼ tsp. salt, and remaining ¼ tsp. pepper.
6. Serve fish in corn tortillas with the cucumber relish, cilantro, cabbage, and avocado.
7. Serve lime wedges on the side.
8. Enjoy!

# Roasted Zucchini Lasagna

**Serves 8**

**332 Calories,** 11.9g Fat, 22.8g Carbs, 10.4g Sugar, 5.8g Fiber, 35.8g Protein

For the "noodles":

2 large zucchini, peeled and sliced lengthwise into ¼-inch noodle-like strips

Salt and pepper to taste

For the meat sauce:

1½ lb. turkey breast

2 onions, chopped

3 cloves garlic, chopped

2 tbsp. olive oil

1 red bell pepper, cored and chopped

1 (16-oz.) package sliced mushrooms

1 (10-oz.) package frozen chopped spinach

1 (28-oz.) can tomato sauce

1 (15-oz.) can diced tomatoes

1 tsp. red pepper flakes (optional)

2 tbsp. Italian seasoning

Salt and pepper, to taste

For the cheese mixture:

2 cups ricotta cheese

2 eggs

3 scallions, chopped

3 cups shredded mozzarella cheese

½ cup grated Parmesan cheese

1. Preheat oven to 425°F. Spray a baking sheet with cooking spray.

For the "noodles":

2. Arrange zucchini slices on baking sheet and season with salt and pepper.

3. Transfer to oven and bake for 5 minutes on each side.

4. Reduce oven temperature to 375°F.

*(continued on next page)*

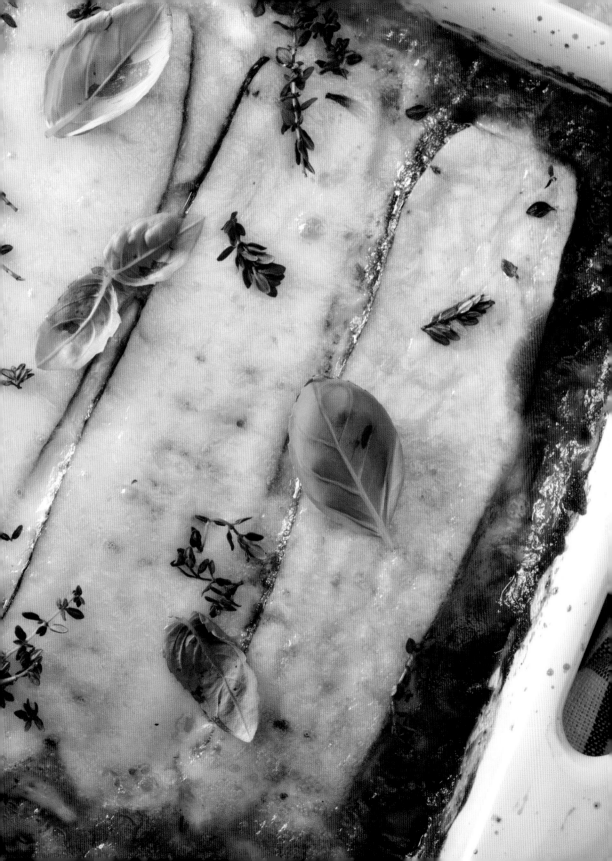

For the meat sauce:

5.  In a large skillet over medium heat, brown turkey, onion, and garlic in olive oil for 5 minutes.

6.  Add red pepper and mushrooms, and cook for 5 minutes.

7.  Add spinach, tomato sauce, diced tomatoes, red pepper flakes, and Italian seasoning, and season with salt and pepper.

8.  Simmer for 5–10 minutes.

For the cheese mixture:

9.  In a bowl, mix together ricotta cheese, eggs, and scallions.

10. Spread one-third of meat sauce in bottom of 9 × 13-inch baking dish.

11. Layer half zucchini slices on top, spread with half ricotta mixture, and sprinkle with one-third of the mozzarella and Parmesan.

12. Repeat the layers one more time.

13. Add the last layer of sauce, then sprinkle remaining mozzarella and Parmesan on top.

14. Cover with foil and bake for 1 hour.

15. Remove foil and bake for another 5–10 minutes, until cheese is browned.

16. Let cool for 10 minutes before serving.

17. Enjoy.

# Pan-Seared Salmon Salad

**Serves 4**

**219 Calories,** 11.2g Fat, 9g Carbs, 4.4g Sugar, 2.2g Fiber, 20g Protein

3 tbsp. balsamic vinegar
1 tbsp. extra virgin olive oil for pan and salmon, divided
1½ tsp. dried basil
1 tsp. Dijon mustard
⅛ tsp. salt
½ cup sliced cherry tomatoes
1 lb. mixed salad greens
1 small onion, minced
4 (3-oz.) salmon fillets, skin removed
1 tsp. Italian seasoning
Lemon wedges, for serving

1. In a large bowl, whisk together balsamic vinegar, ½ tbsp. of the oil, basil, mustard, and salt until smooth.

2. Place tomatoes and greens in the bowl and toss to coat with the dressing. Set aside.

3. Coat a medium skillet lightly with remaining ½ tbsp. olive oil.

4. Add onion. Cook over medium-high heat for 5–7 minutes, or until soft.

5. Remove to a plate to cool.

6. Wipe out skillet with a paper towel.

7. Coat with olive oil and place over high heat.

8. Lightly coat salmon with olive oil and sprinkle with Italian seasoning.

9. Add the salmon to skillet and cook for 3 minutes on each side, or until it flakes easily.

10. Remove from heat and cut fillets into medium-size pieces.

*(continued on next page)*

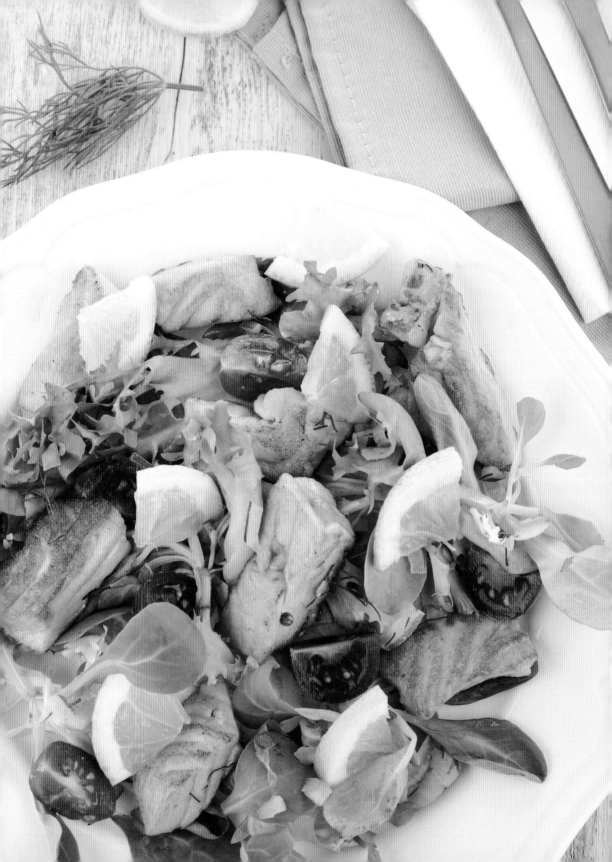

11. Add onions and salmon to salad bowl.

12. Toss gently to mix.

13. Spoon salad onto four plates.

14. Serve with lemon wedges.

15. Dig in!

# Santa Fe Black Beans with Chicken

**Serves 2**

**400 Calories,** 18.7g Fat, 25.3g Carbs, 0g Sugar, 7.6g Fiber, 33.2g Protein

1 tsp. ground cumin
Kosher salt and black pepper to taste
¼ tsp. cayenne pepper
4 small chicken drumsticks
2 tbsp. olive oil
1 cup canned black beans, rinsed and drained
Lime wedges

1. Combine cumin, salt and pepper, and cayenne pepper in a small bowl and rub on chicken.
2. In a large skillet, heat oil over medium heat.
3. Sauté chicken for 4 minutes per side, or until no longer pink.
4. Remove from heat.
5. Heat up black beans in a microwave-safe bowl or in a small pot on stove top.
6. Divide beans between two plates and top with drumsticks and lime wedges.
7. Serve immediately.
8. Enjoy!

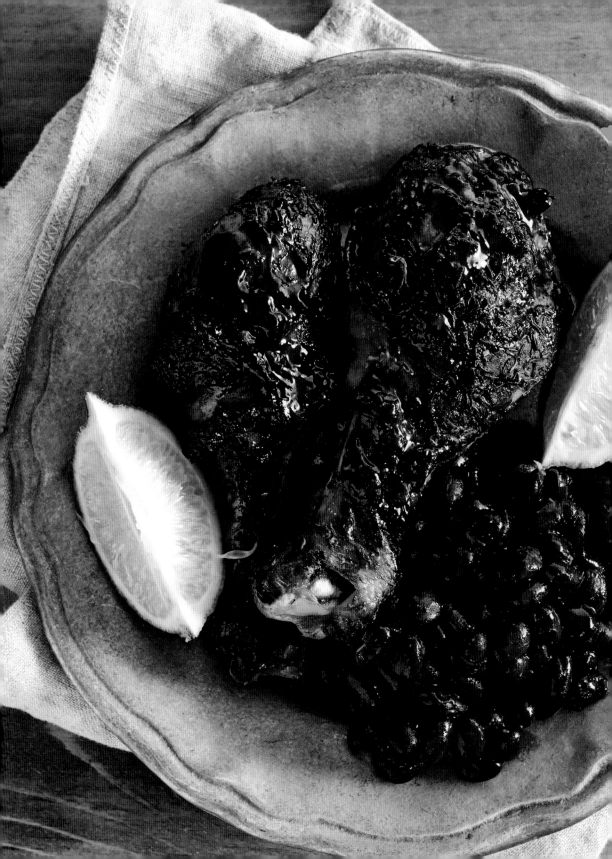

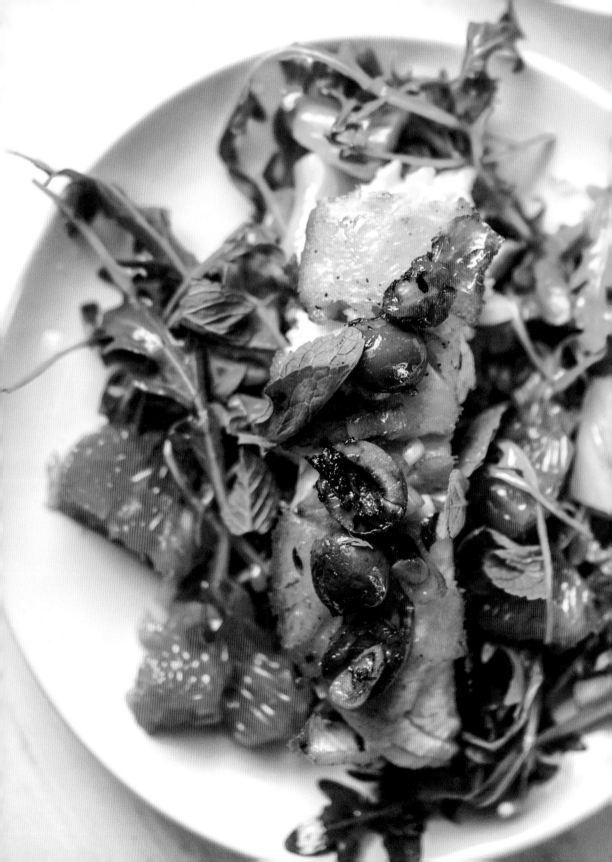

# Grilled Tilapia Grapefruit Salad

**Serves 4**

**260 Calories,** 16.6g Fat, 7.1g Carbs, 5.4g Sugar, 0.8g Fiber, 18g Protein

4 tbsp. olive oil, divided, plus more if needed

4 (3-oz.) tilapia fillets

¾ tsp. kosher salt, divided

½ tsp. black pepper, divided

2 tbsp. fresh lime juice

1 tbsp. Dijon mustard

2 tsp. honey

6 cups arugula, thick stems removed

2 heads endive, sliced

1 grapefruit, supremed

2 tbsp. sliced green olives

1. Heat 2 tbsp. oil in a nonstick pan over medium-high heat.

2. Season tilapia fillets with ½ tsp. salt and ¼ tsp. pepper.

3. Add fillets to pan and cook for 2–3 minutes per side until cooked through (adding more oil to pan, if needed).

4. Remove from pan and let cool.

5. In a large bowl, whisk together lime juice, mustard, honey, remaining 2 tbsp. oil, remaining ¼ tsp. salt, and remaining ¼ tsp. pepper.

6. Add arugula, endive, grapefruit, and olives.

7. Toss lightly.

8. Plate salad and top with tilapia fillets.

9. *Buen appetit*!

# Asparagus Cauliflower Pizza

**Serves 1**

**331 Calories,** 5.2g Fat, 42.8g Carbs, 20.8g Sugar, 15.1g Fiber, 43.4g Protein

For the crust:
2½ cups grated cauliflower
1 large egg
¾ cup fat-free mozzarella, divided
2 tbsp. grated Parmesan cheese
Pinch of salt

For the toppings:
¼ cup marinara
½ medium cucumber, sliced
10 asparagus stalks
30 basil leaves
5 oregano leaves

1. Preheat oven to 425°F. Line a rimmed baking sheet with parchment paper.

For the crust:

2. Place the grated cauliflower in a large bowl and microwave for 7–8 minutes or until soft.

3. Remove and let cool.

4. In the bowl with cauliflower, mix in egg, mozzarella, Parmesan cheese, and salt. Combine well.

5. Pat into a 10-inch round on the prepared baking sheet.

6. Spray lightly with nonstick spray and bake for 10–15 minutes or until golden.

For the toppings:

7. Top the pizza crust with sauce, cucumber, and asparagus.

8. Bake in the oven until crust becomes bubbly, about another 10 minutes.

9. Remove from oven and top with basil and oregano leaves.

10. Slice and serve.

11. *Buon appetito!*

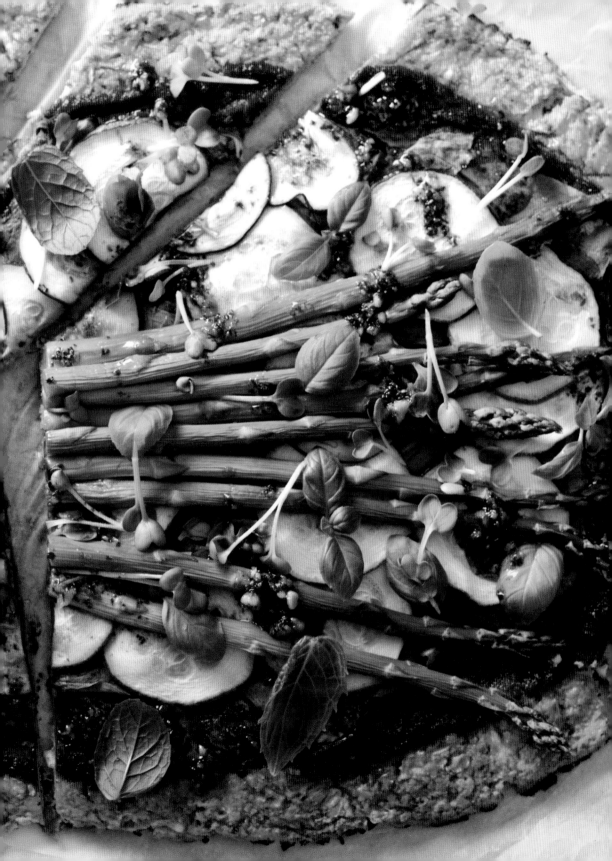

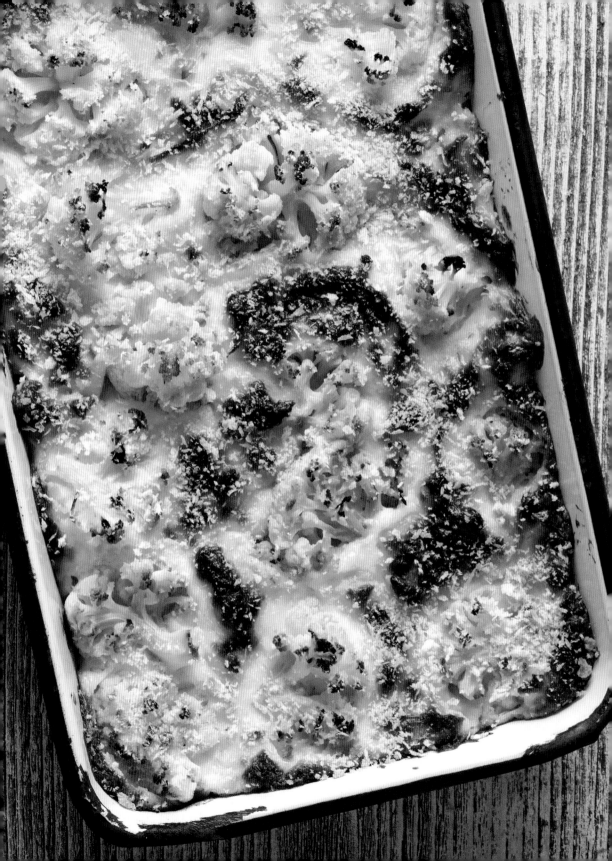

# Baked Cauliflower Casserole

**Serves 6**

**250 Calories,** 15g Fat, 16g Carbs, 8g Sugar, 3g Fiber, 13g Protein

1 large cauliflower (leaves cut off), broken into pieces
¼ cup milk
4 tbsp. whole-wheat flour
3 tbsp. butter
2 cups grated cheddar cheese
2–3 tbsp. whole-wheat breadcrumbs

1. Preheat oven to 425°F.
2. Bring a large saucepan of water to a boil.
3. Add cauliflower and cook for 5 minutes, or until tender.
4. Drain cauliflower and add to an oven-safe baking dish.
5. Place saucepan back on the heat and add milk, flour, and butter.
6. Whisk as the butter melts and mixture comes to a boil—the flour will disappear and the sauce will begin to thicken.
7. Whisk for 2 minutes while the sauce bubbles and becomes thick.
8. Turn off heat and stir in most of the cheese.
9. Pour mixture over cauliflower.
10. Top with the remaining cheese and breadcrumbs.
11. Bake for 20 minutes, or until bubbling.
12. Dig in!

# Chicken Supreme Salad

**Serves 4**

**194 Calories,** 8.2g Fat, 6.8g Carbs, 3.9g Sugar, 0.6g Fiber, 21.2g Protein

4 (3-oz.) chicken breasts
1 tbsp. extra virgin olive oil
6 tbsp. balsamic vinegar, divided
6 tsp. minced garlic
4 cups mixed greens
½ cup shredded Parmesan cheese

1. In a pan over medium heat, cook chicken breasts in olive oil, 4 tbsp. balsamic vinegar, and garlic.

2. Remove from heat when cooked through and no longer pink.

3. In a large bowl, toss together mixed greens, Parmesan cheese, and remaining 2 tbsp. balsamic vinegar.

4. Divide among four plates and top each salad with a balsamic chicken breast.

5. Enjoy!

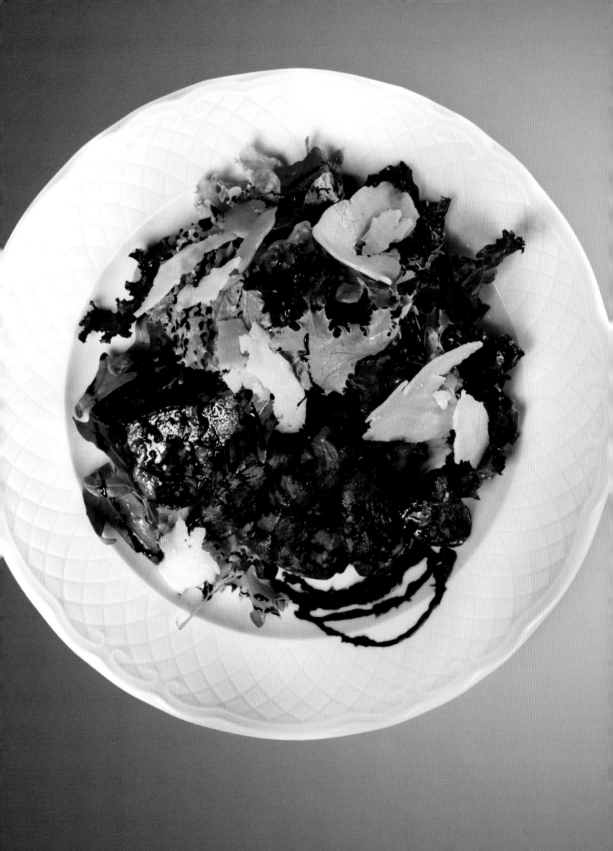

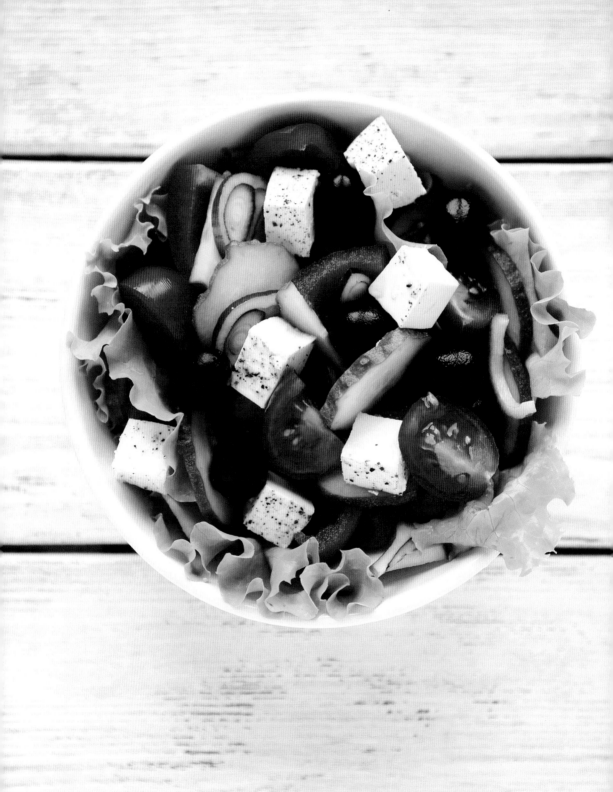

# Garden Greek Salad

**Serves 4**

**312 Calories,** 28.9g Fat, 10g Carbs, 2.2g Sugar, 0.8g Fiber, 6g Protein

1 cup cherry tomatoes, halved
1 red onion, thinly sliced
1 cucumber, sliced
½ cup Kalamata black olives
2 (4-oz.) slices Greek feta
4 tbsp. extra virgin olive oil
3 tbsp. red wine vinegar
1 tsp. dried oregano, crushed
Salt and pepper, to taste

1. In a large bowl, combine tomatoes, onion, cucumber, olives, and feta.
2. In a small bowl, whisk together olive oil, vinegar, and oregano.
3. Pour over salad and season with salt and pepper.
4. Enjoy!

# Guilt-Free Zucchini Pasta

**Serves 2**

**222 Calories,** 18.6g Fat, 25.8g Carbs, 7g Sugar, 2.6g Fiber, 5.5g Protein

2 tbsp. olive oil
3 cloves garlic, minced
½ onion, sliced
1 large zucchini, spiraled or grated
½ cup chopped cherry tomatoes
¼ cup cubed feta
Salt and pepper, to taste

1. In a medium pan over low heat, add olive oil.

2. Let heat for 1 minute.

3. Add minced garlic to oil.

4. Use a spoon or spatula to stir garlic to keep it from sticking to the pan and burning.

5. When garlic becomes fragrant, add onion and stir.

6. Cook until onions become soft and slightly brown, 4–5 minutes.

7. Place zucchini "noodles" in a large bowl.

8. Pour onion-garlic mixture over zucchini, add tomatoes and cheese, and toss gently to combine.

9. Season with salt and pepper.

10. Dig in!

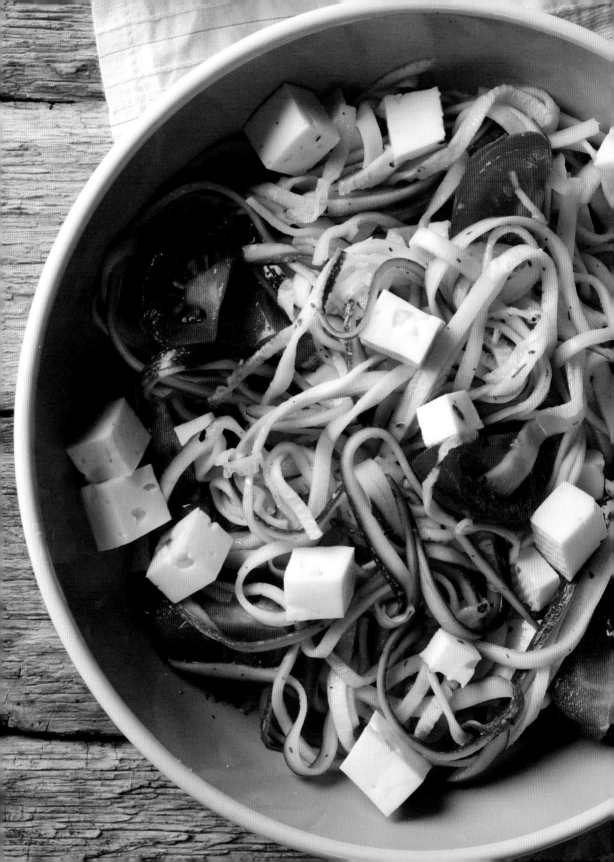

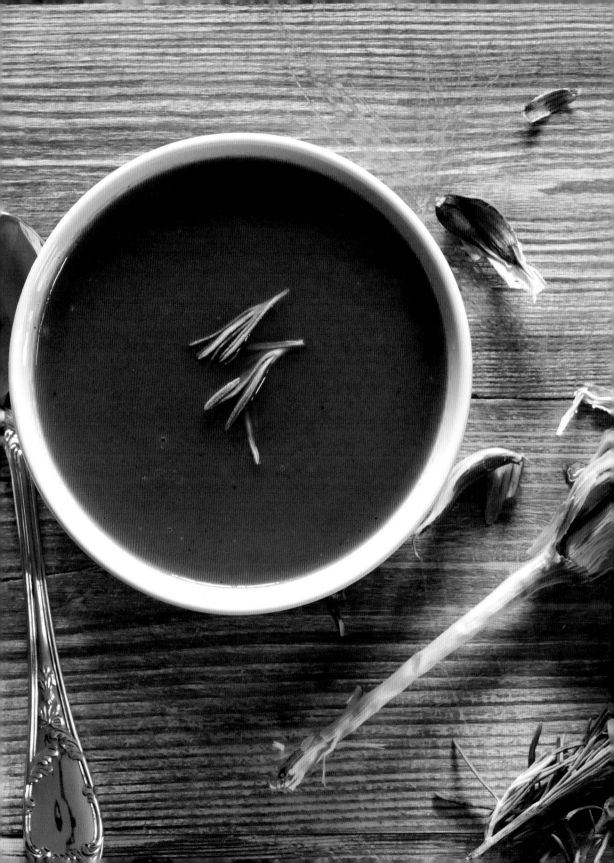

# Organic Artichoke Tomato Soup

**Serves 4**

**342 Calories,** 30.6g Fat, 35.15g Carbs, 16.6g Sugar, 4.2g Fiber, 20.8g Protein

1 (28-oz.) can whole tomatoes in puree
3 tbsp. unsalted butter
1 cup diced sweet onion
¾ cup thinly sliced scallion, white and green parts
2 cloves garlic, minced
2 tbsp. tomato paste
3 tbsp. all-purpose flour
1½ cups low-sodium chicken broth
2½ cups milk
1 (9-oz.) package frozen artichoke hearts, thawed and roughly chopped
2 tsp. kosher salt
1½ cups shredded sharp white cheddar cheese
¼ cup heavy cream

1. In a large bowl, pour in tomatoes and puree.
2. Break up into small pieces with a wooden spoon or kitchen shears and set aside.
3. In a 6-qt. pot over medium heat, melt butter.
4. Add onion, scallion, and garlic.
5. Cook, stirring occasionally, until onions are just soft, 3–5 minutes.
6. Add tomato paste and flour.
7. Stir for about 1 minute to cook the flour and heat through.
8. Stir in broth, milk, artichokes, salt, and tomatoes in puree.
9. Bring the soup to a simmer, making sure not to boil.
10. Cover pot and simmer, stirring occasionally, for 15–20 minutes to meld flavors.
11. When done, add cheese and cream, stirring until cheese is melted.
12. *Buen appetit!*

# Spaghetti Squash Pasta

**Serves 8**

**300 Calories,** 14.1g Fat, 37.4g Carbs, 26.6g Sugar, 9g Fiber, 7g Protein

2 whole spaghetti squash
¼ cup extra virgin olive oil
Salt and pepper, to taste
4 cups marinara sauce
Finely grated Parmesan cheese
8 basil leaves (optional)

1. Preheat oven to 450°F.
2. Line a baking sheet with aluminum foil.
3. Cut squashes in half and remove seeds.
4. Season with olive oil, salt, and pepper.
5. Place squash halves flesh-side down on prepared baking sheet.
6. Roast for 30–40 minutes, or until fully cooked.
7. Remove from oven and let cool until you can handle it.
8. In a medium pot over low heat, heat marinara sauce.
9. When squash is cool enough to touch, use a large spoon to scrape the strands out.
10. Plate spaghetti squash "noodles" and top with warmed marinara.
11. Garnish with a little sprinkle of Parmesan cheese and a basil leaf, if desired.
12. Dig in!

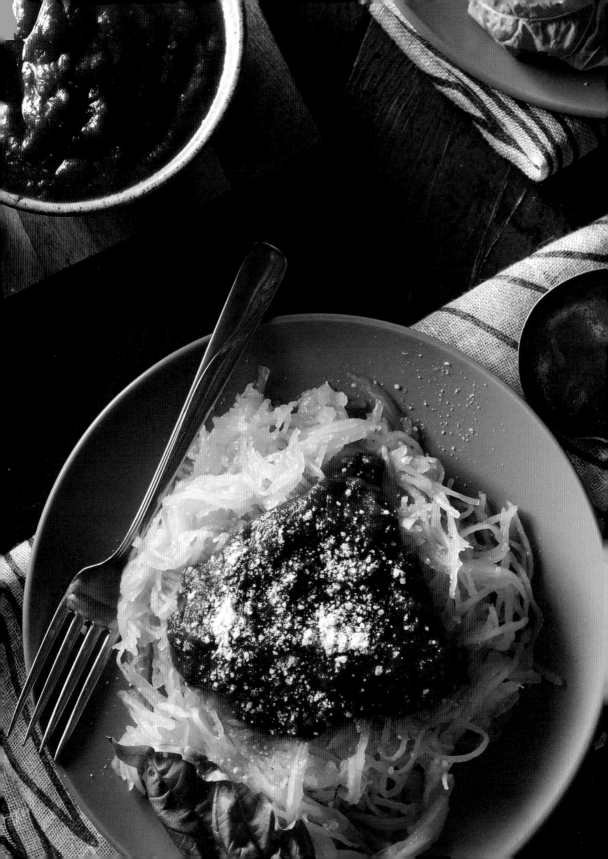

# 10 Tiny and Full™ Dessert Recipes

t's time to indulge!

I am so excited to introduce to you ten oh-so-delicious desserts! Mmm mmm mmm. Use these anytime you need a sweet treat at the end of the night. They are great to share with friends and family!

Take note of calorie counts and either adjust portions or reduce snacks throughout the day to make sure you stay within your calorie goal.

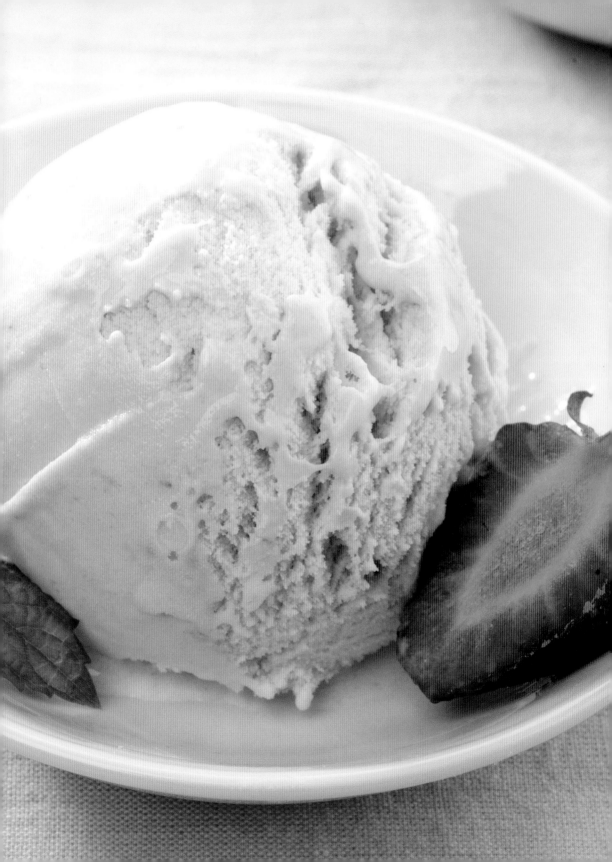

# Banana Berry Ice Cream

**Serves 2**

**96 Calories,** 1g Fat, 22.8g Carbs, 12.1g Sugar, 2.8g Fiber, 1.2g Protein

1½ medium bananas, peeled, sliced, and frozen until solid
⅓ cup chopped frozen strawberries
2 tbsp. cream

1. Place frozen bananas in a blender.
2. Mix until they are the consistency of soft serve ice cream.
3. Add strawberries and cream and blend until smooth.
4. Transfer mixture to a freezer container and freeze until solid.
5. Serve when completely frozen.
6. Enjoy!

# Cocoa Bean Brownies

**Makes 16**

**[Per Square] 112 Calories,** 4.4g Fat, 18.5g Carbs, 11g Sugar, 3.1g Fiber, 2.8g Protein

1 (14-oz.) can black beans, drained and rinsed
2 large eggs
½ cup unsweetened applesauce
15 small dates, pitted (½ cup packed)
2 tbsp. brewed coffee (optional)
1 tsp. pure vanilla extract
½ cup cocoa powder
¼ tsp. salt
½ tsp. baking soda
¾ cup dark chocolate chips, divided

1.  Preheat oven to 350°F.
2.  Line an 8 × 8-inch baking dish with parchment paper and spray with cooking spray.
3.  Add all ingredients, except chocolate chips, to a blender.
4.  Blend until smooth.
5.  Add ½ cup chocolate chips and stir to mix.
6.  Pour batter into baking dish and top with remaining ¼ cup chocolate chips.
7.  Bake for 30 minutes.
8.  Remove from oven and let brownies cool completely.
9.  Cut into 16 squares and serve.
10. Enjoy.

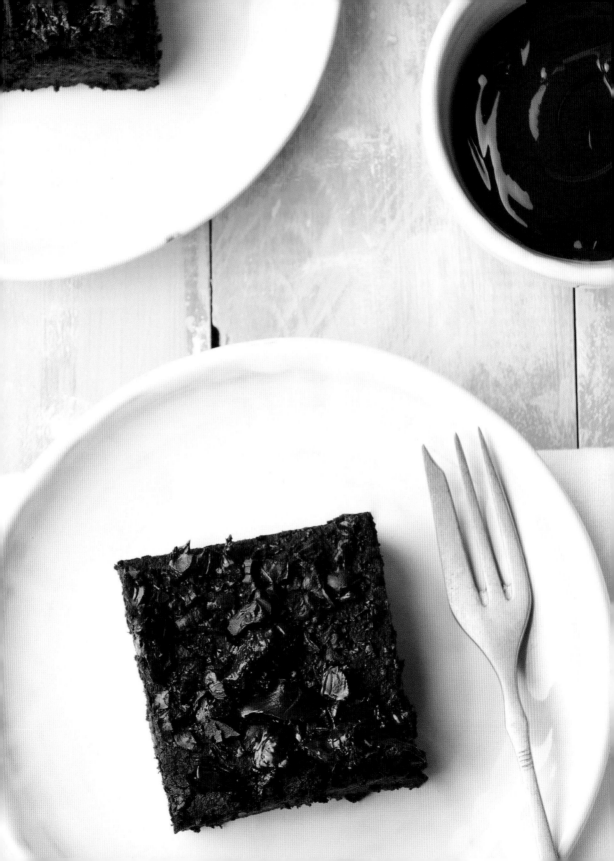

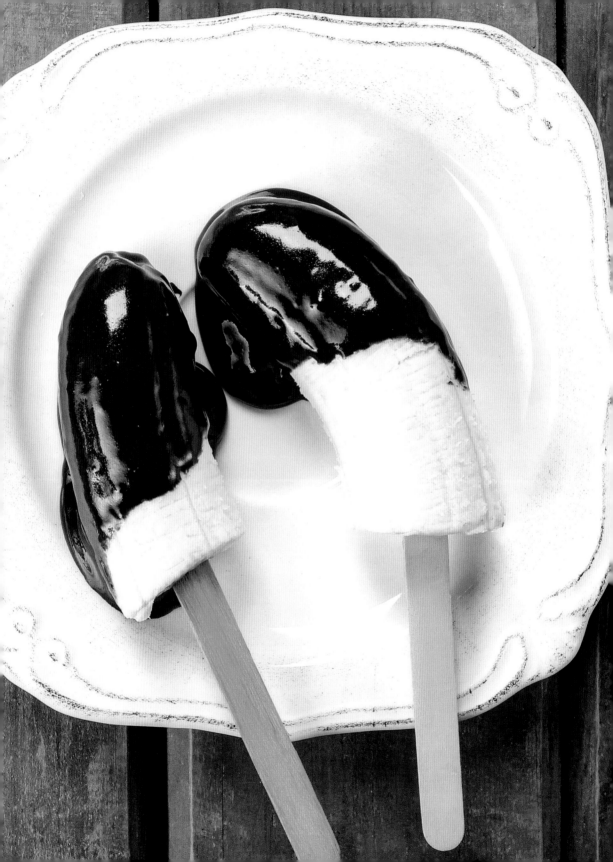

# Carob Chocolate Bananas

**Makes 4**

**[Per banana] 253 Calories,** 10.3g Fat, 36.2g Carbs, 27g Sugar, 7.2g Fiber, 6.4g Protein

2 bananas
3 tbsp. unsweetened almond milk
1 (6-oz.) bag carob chips (you can also use semisweet morsels)

1. Peel bananas and cut in half.
2. Push ice pop sticks into bottoms.
3. Add almond milk and carob chips to a pot and allow to melt, stirring as it goes.
4. Dip bananas in chocolate, holding onto stick.
5. Refrigerate for a minimum of 3 hours, then serve.
6. Sit back, relax, and enjoy.

# Chocolate Avocado Mousse Cupcakes

**Makes 12**

**[Per Cupcake] 230 Calories,** 13.6g Fat, 28.3g Carbs, 16.1g Sugar, 4.7g Fiber, 2.9g Protein

For the cupcakes:
1 cup unsweetened almond milk
1 tsp. apple cider vinegar
¾ cup sugar
⅓ cup canola oil
1½ tsp. vanilla extract
1 cup white whole-wheat flour
⅓ cup unsweetened cocoa powder
¾ tsp. baking soda
½ tsp. baking powder
¼ tsp. sea salt

For the frosting:
2 ripe avocados
¼ cup unsweetened cocoa powder
3 tbsp. pure maple syrup
½ tsp. vanilla extract

1. Preheat oven to 350°F.
2. Line a muffin tin with 12 cupcake liners.

For the cupcakes:

3. In a bowl, whisk together almond milk and apple cider vinegar, and set aside for a few minutes so that the milk curdles.
4. Beat in sugar, oil, and vanilla until it becomes foamy.

*(continued on next page)*

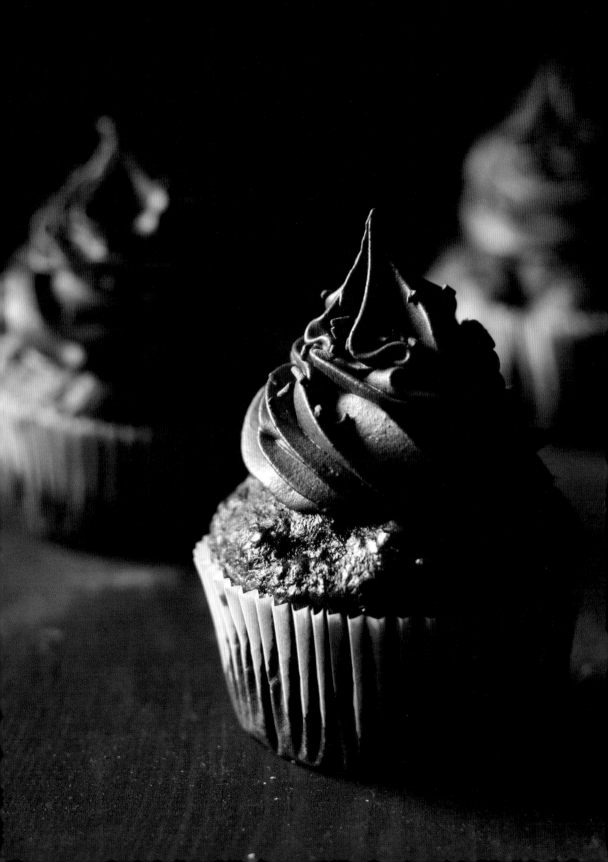

5. In a separate bowl, mix together flour, cocoa powder, baking soda, baking powder, and salt.

6. Slowly mix dry ingredients into wet ingredients until smooth.

7. Pour batter evenly among cupcake liners.

8. Bake for 18–25 minutes, or until a toothpick inserted into the center comes out clean.

9. Remove from oven, and after a few minutes, move cupcakes to a cooling rack.

For the frosting:

10. While the cupcakes bake, make the frosting.

11. Scoop out avocado flesh and place in a food processor.

12. Add cocoa powder, maple syrup, and vanilla, and blend until smooth.

13. Frost the cooled cupcakes.

14. Enjoy.

# Flourless Chocolate Cookie Dough Bites

**Makes 32**

**[Per Bite] 66 Calories,** 3.8g Fat, 7.9g Carbs, 4.2g Sugar, 1.1g Fiber, 1.3g Protein

1½ cups chickpeas, rinsed and drained

2 tbsp. molasses

1 tbsp. agave nectar or honey

4 tbsp. almond butter

1 tbsp. pure vanilla extract

1–2 tsp. ground cinnamon

½ tsp. ground ginger

⅛ tsp. baking soda

Salt to taste

½ cup uncooked oats

¾ cup semisweet chocolate chips, divided

2 tbsp. coconut oil

1. In a food processor or blender, mix together chickpeas, molasses, agave nectar, almond butter, vanilla, cinnamon, ginger, baking soda, and salt until smooth.

2. Scoop out contents into a medium bowl.

3. Add oats and ¼ cup chocolate chips. Mix well.

4. Line a baking sheet with aluminum foil.

5. Form small balls from dough and place on baking sheet.

6. Freeze for about 15 minutes, or until hard.

7. While dough is freezing, melt remaining ½ cup chocolate chips and coconut oil in a microwave-safe bowl in 20-second increments, stirring in between until smooth.

*(continued on next page)*

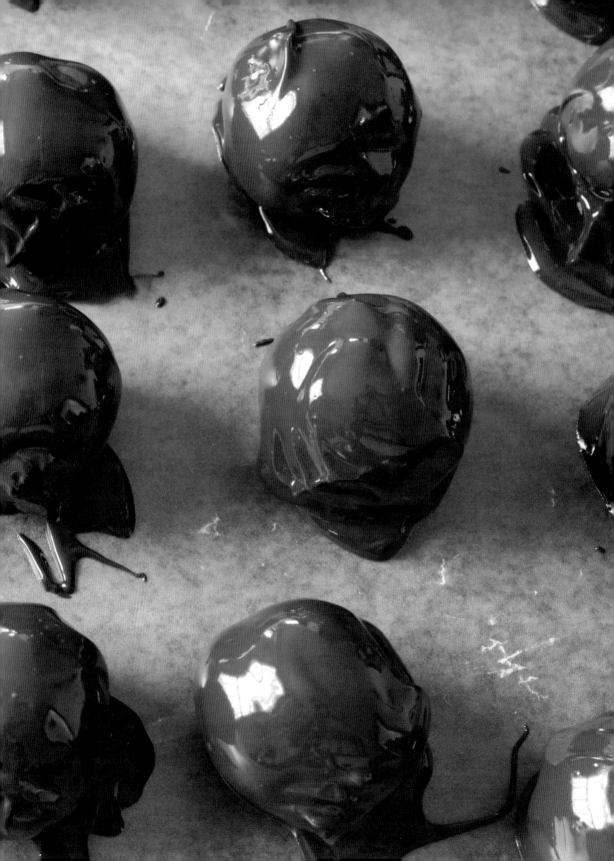

8.  Remove the dough from freezer and dip each ball into melted chocolate.

9.  Place back on baking sheet.

10. Put bites back into the freezer or refrigerator until chocolate is hard.

11. When ready to eat, remove from freezer and thaw for a few minutes.

12. Enjoy.

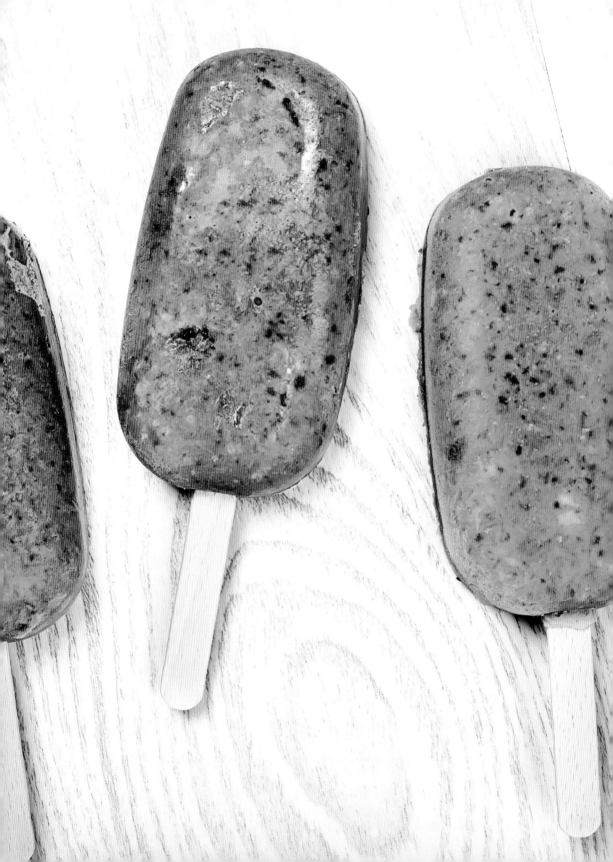

# Strawberry Yogurt Ice Pops

**Makes 6**

**[Per Ice Pop] 50** Calories, 0.3g Fat, 11g Carbs, 8.7g Sugar, 2g Fiber, 4.2g Protein

35 medium strawberries, hulled and roughly chopped
2 tbsp. sugar
1 tsp. lemon juice
4 oz. fat-free Greek yogurt
½ cup water

1. Place all ingredients in a blender and blend until smooth.
2. Pour mixture into ice pop molds and freeze for 4 hours.
3. Enjoy!

# Peanut Butter Fudge

**Makes 8**

**[Per Square] 137 Calories,** 11.5g Fat, 6.5g Carbs, 4.5g Sugar, 1g Fiber, 4.1g Protein

½ cup peanut butter
2 tbsp. coconut oil, softened
2 tbsp. maple syrup
¼ tsp. pure vanilla extract
¼ tsp. salt

1. In a large bowl, mix together all ingredients until well combined. (You can microwave the mixture for about 15 seconds if it is hard to mix.)

2. Line an 8 × 8-inch baking pan with parchment paper.

3. Pour fudge into pan.

4. Place in freezer for 30–40 minutes.

5. Once fudge has completely hardened, remove from pan and let sit for 5 minutes.

6. Use a sharp knife to cut fudge into 8 squares.

7. Serve or re-freeze until ready to serve.

8. Enjoy.

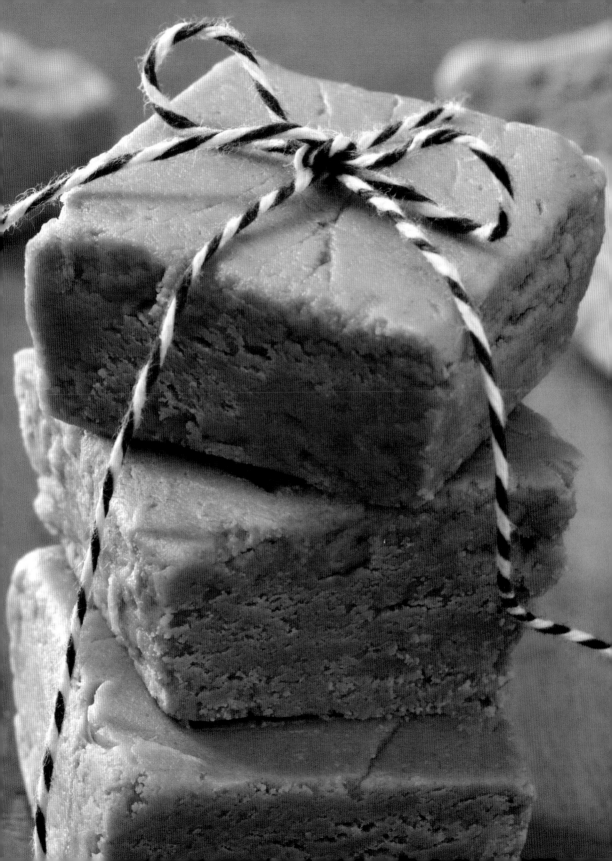

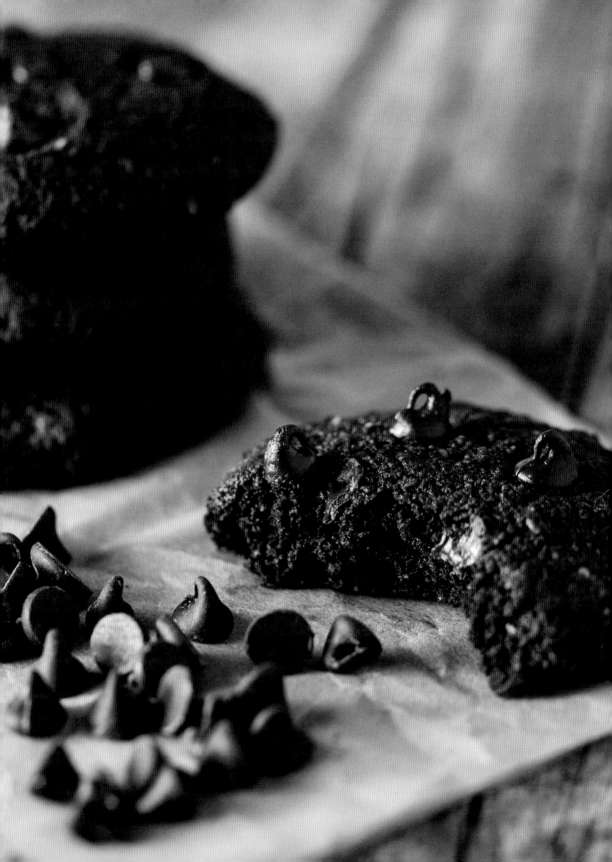

# Sam's 20-Calorie Mint Chocolate Cookie

**Makes 10**

**[Per Cookie] 20 Calories,** 1g Fat, 2.8g Carbs, 0.1g Sugar, 1.1g Fiber, 1.1g Protein

1 (8-oz.) bag shirataki noodles
1 tbsp. lemon juice
3 tbsp. cocoa powder
½ tsp. baking powder
2 tsp. stevia powder
Dash of salt
⅛ tsp. mint extract
120 unsweetened chocolate chips

1. Preheat oven to 375°F.
2. Lightly grease a cookie sheet.
3. Rinse shirataki noodles in a strainer with hot water.
4. Sprinkle with lemon juice and let sit for a minute, then rinse again in hot water. Drain well.
5. Add noodles to a large pan and cook over high heat until they lose translucency, stirring often.
6. Remove from heat and let cool.
7. Add to a food processor.
8. Blend until mixture has the consistency of gel.
9. Quickly add cocoa powder, baking powder, stevia powder, salt, mint extract, and chocolate chips.
10. Blend well. (If dough is on the runny side, stick it in the fridge for 1 hour.)
11. When ready, drop spoonfuls of dough onto prepared cookie sheet.
12. Bake for 10 minutes.
13. Let cool for a few minutes.
14. Enjoy!

# Watermelon Lover's Pizza

**Serves 12**

**[Per Wedge] 26 Calories,** 0.9g Fat, 6.5g Carbs, 4.5g Sugar, 0.5g Fiber, 0.4g Protein

1 banana, sliced
¼ cup blueberries
2 (1-inch thick) round watermelon slices, 8–9-inch diameter
2 tbsp. honey
2 tbsp. lime juice
1 tsp. finely grated lime zest
2 tbsp. chopped fresh mint

1. Arrange banana slices and blueberries on watermelon rounds.
2. Cut each round into 6 wedges.
3. In a small bowl, whisk together honey, lime juice, and lime zest.
4. Drizzle mixture over watermelon and garnish with mint.
5. Enjoy!

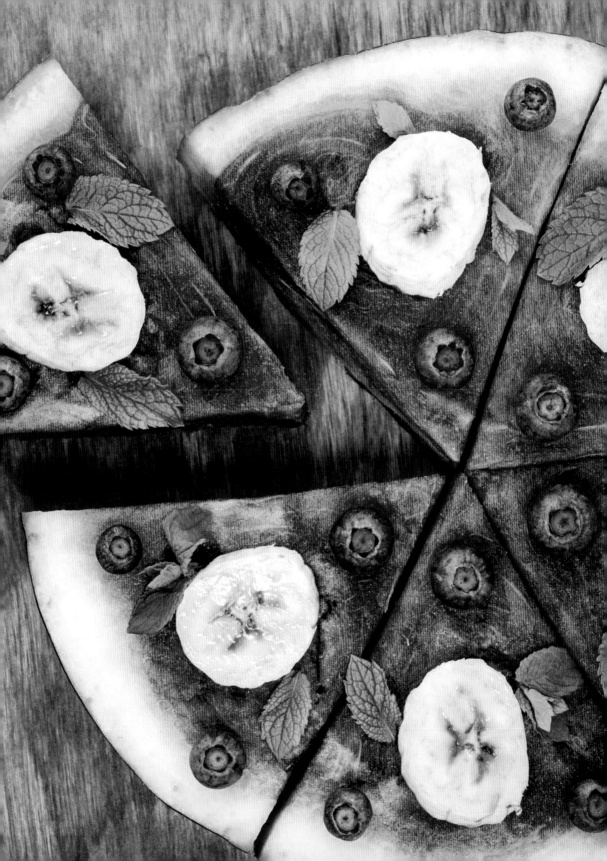

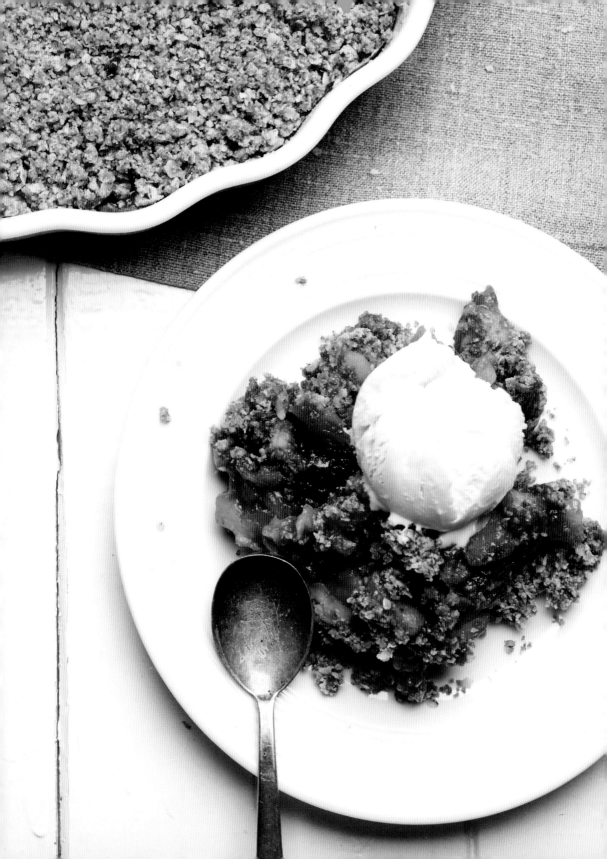

# Apple Crisp

**Serves 9**

**79 Calories,** 0.4g Fat, 19.2g Carbs, 11.6g Sugar, 4.7g Fiber, 0.7g Protein

For the apples:
3 medium apples, cored and thinly sliced
1 tsp. ground cinnamon
½ tsp. ground cloves
¼ cup applesauce

For the topping:
1 cup quick oats
1 tsp. pure vanilla extract
½ tsp. ground cinnamon
¼ cup brown sugar
2 tbsp. applesauce
1 cup fat-free Cool Whip

1. Preheat oven to 325°F.

For the apples:

2. In a bowl, mix together apples, cinnamon, cloves, and applesauce.

3. Place mixture into 9-inch (square or round) baking dish.

For the topping:

4. In a small bowl, mix oats, vanilla, cinnamon, brown sugar, and applesauce until crumbly.

5. Sprinkle topping over apples.

6. Bake until apples are soft and topping is golden brown, about 30 minutes.

7. Let cool slightly.

8. Serve with a dollop of Cool Whip.

9. Dig in!

# Conclusion

You've reached the end of the book! I want to take this moment to thank you for reading and I hope you now know that you deserve to be Tiny, but don't have to suffer getting there.

If you have yet to start your 12-week challenge to kick off your new Tiny and Full™ lifestyle, I encourage you to turn to the meal planners in Chapter 4 and get started today.

If you're reading this and you have completed your 12-week challenge, congratulations! I want to invite you to share this message with your friends and family, as well as share your success with me personally. Please visit TinyandFull.com and tag me on social media (@TinyandFull and #TinyandFull). Share your stories of success and your favorite Wake Up Vegan™ meals, and be inspired by all of the others following this lifestyle. I can't wait to find out how you did and how you will continue on this journey!

No matter what stage you are at, I encourage you to be an ambassador for Tiny and Full™ so we can change the world together! Let's do this!

We are who we hang around, proximity is power. Use the next few pages to immerse yourself into the Tiny and Full culture, for incredible motivation and inspiration from my Tiny and Full Ambassadors. They will inspire you to live this lifestyle. Teachers, yoga instructors, business people, busy moms, brides to be, even professional athletes. These are all busy, everyday people just like you who have sent photos in to me, including myself! Remember to surround yourself with people who will empower you to succeed to keep you Tiny and Full.

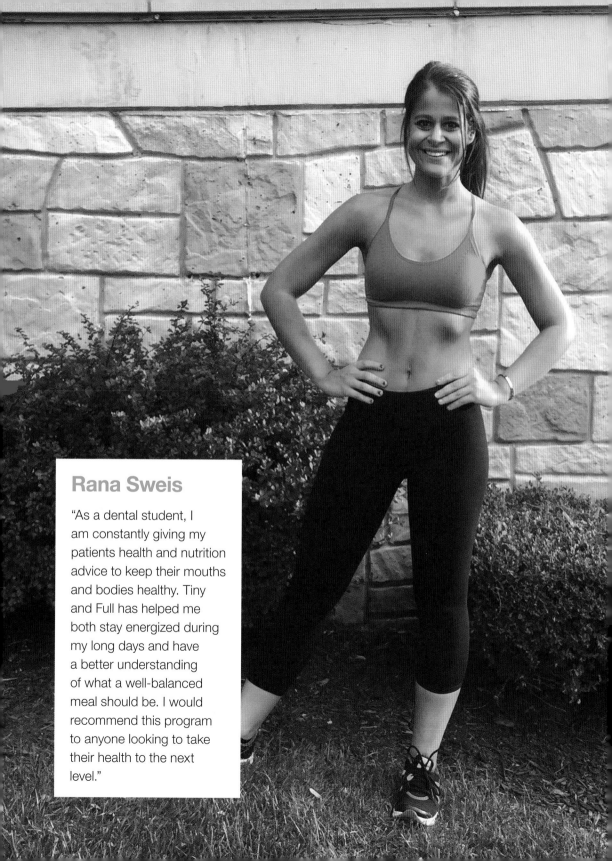

## Rana Sweis

"As a dental student, I am constantly giving my patients health and nutrition advice to keep their mouths and bodies healthy. Tiny and Full has helped me both stay energized during my long days and have a better understanding of what a well-balanced meal should be. I would recommend this program to anyone looking to take their health to the next level."

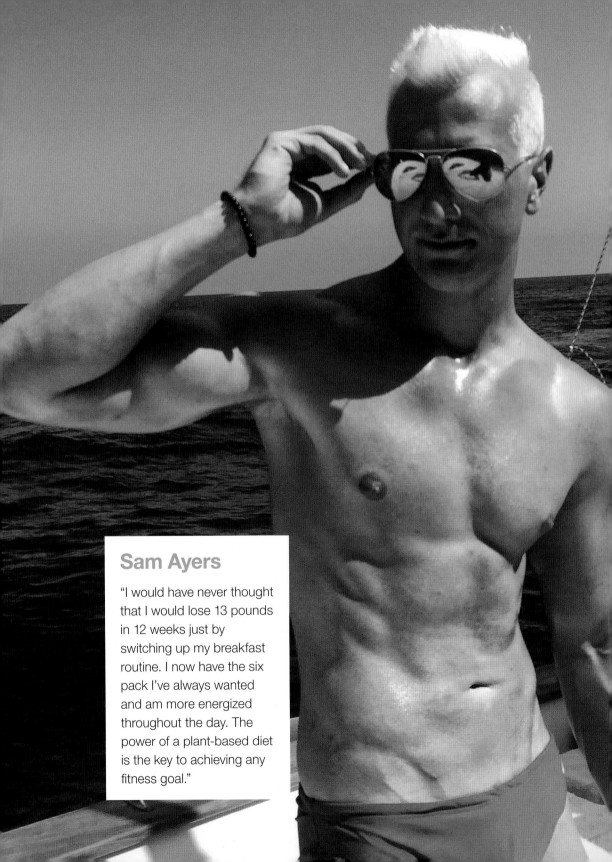

## Sam Ayers

"I would have never thought that I would lose 13 pounds in 12 weeks just by switching up my breakfast routine. I now have the six pack I've always wanted and am more energized throughout the day. The power of a plant-based diet is the key to achieving any fitness goal."

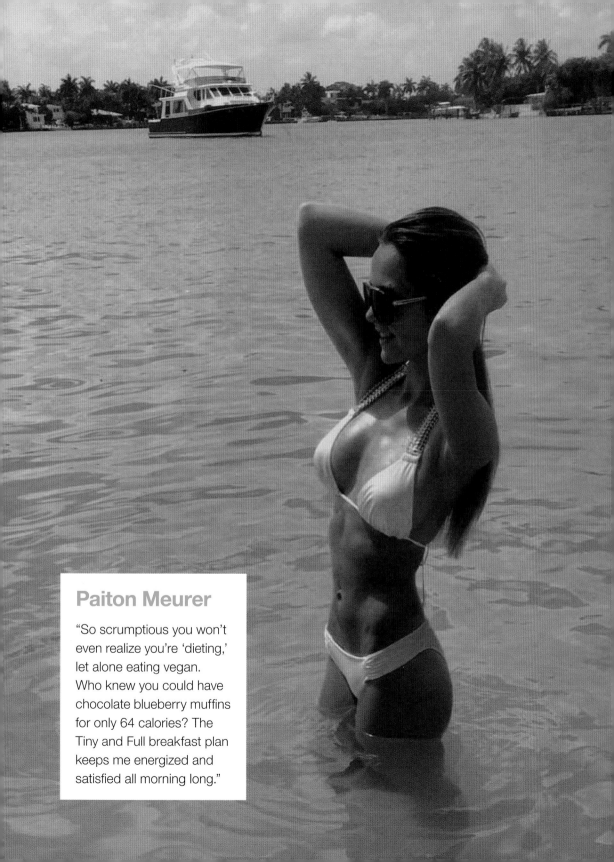

## Paiton Meurer

"So scrumptious you won't even realize you're 'dieting,' let alone eating vegan. Who knew you could have chocolate blueberry muffins for only 64 calories? The Tiny and Full breakfast plan keeps me energized and satisfied all morning long."

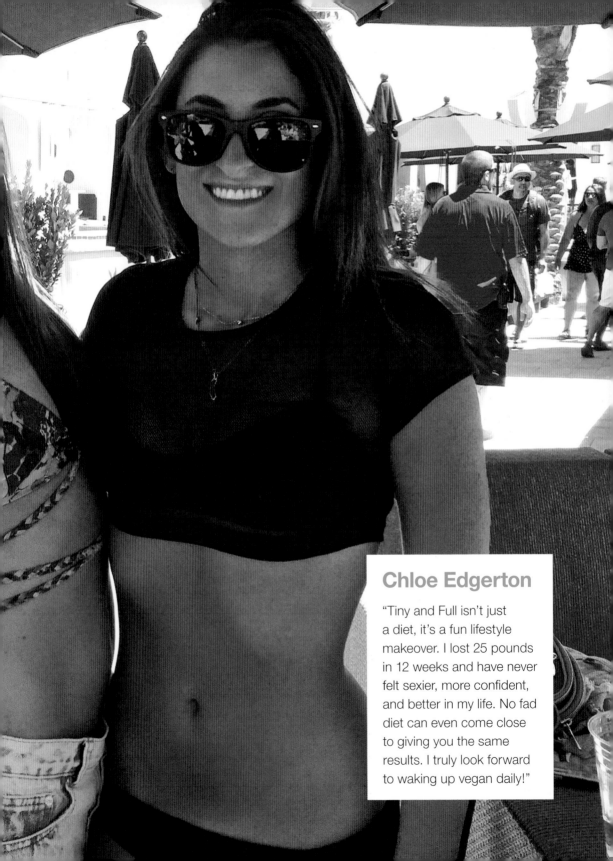

## Chloe Edgerton

"Tiny and Full isn't just a diet, it's a fun lifestyle makeover. I lost 25 pounds in 12 weeks and have never felt sexier, more confident, and better in my life. No fad diet can even come close to giving you the same results. I truly look forward to waking up vegan daily!"

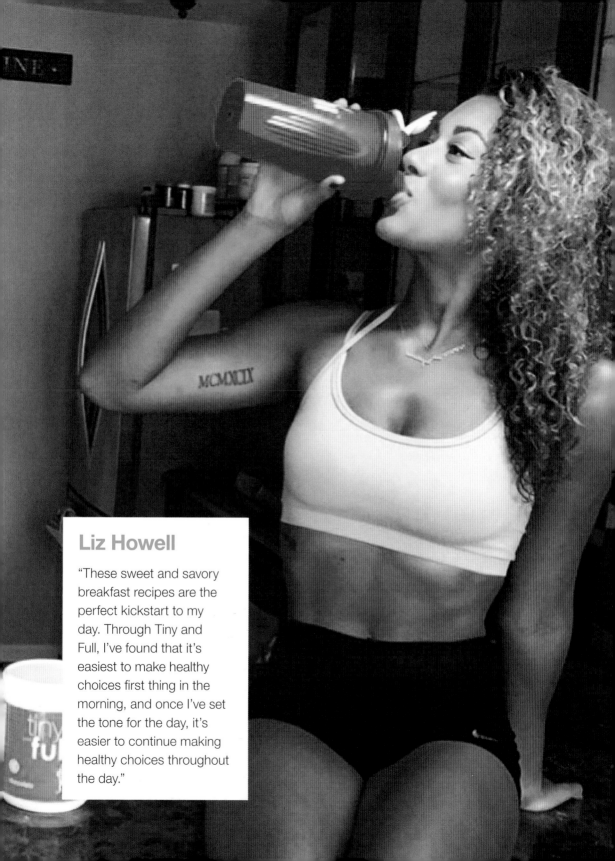

## Liz Howell

"These sweet and savory breakfast recipes are the perfect kickstart to my day. Through Tiny and Full, I've found that it's easiest to make healthy choices first thing in the morning, and once I've set the tone for the day, it's easier to continue making healthy choices throughout the day."

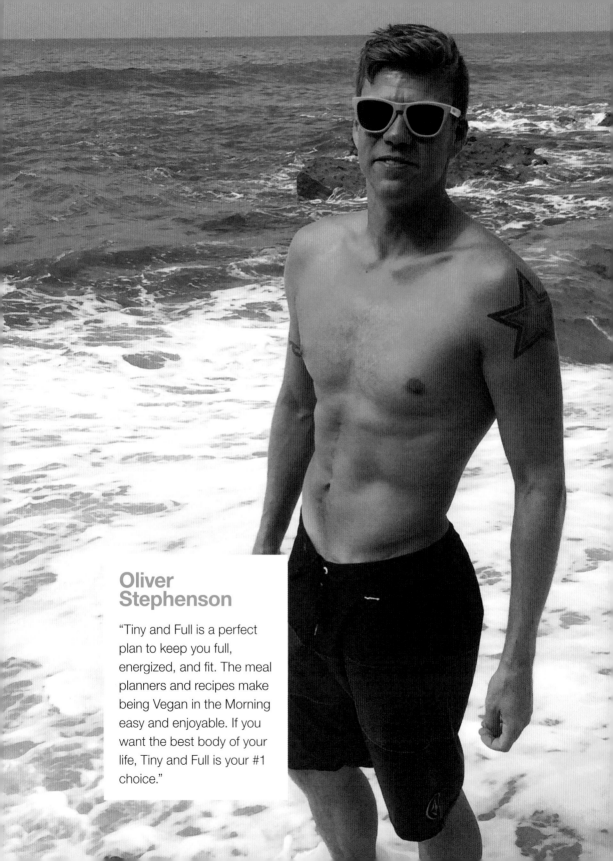

## Oliver Stephenson

"Tiny and Full is a perfect plan to keep you full, energized, and fit. The meal planners and recipes make being Vegan in the Morning easy and enjoyable. If you want the best body of your life, Tiny and Full is your #1 choice."

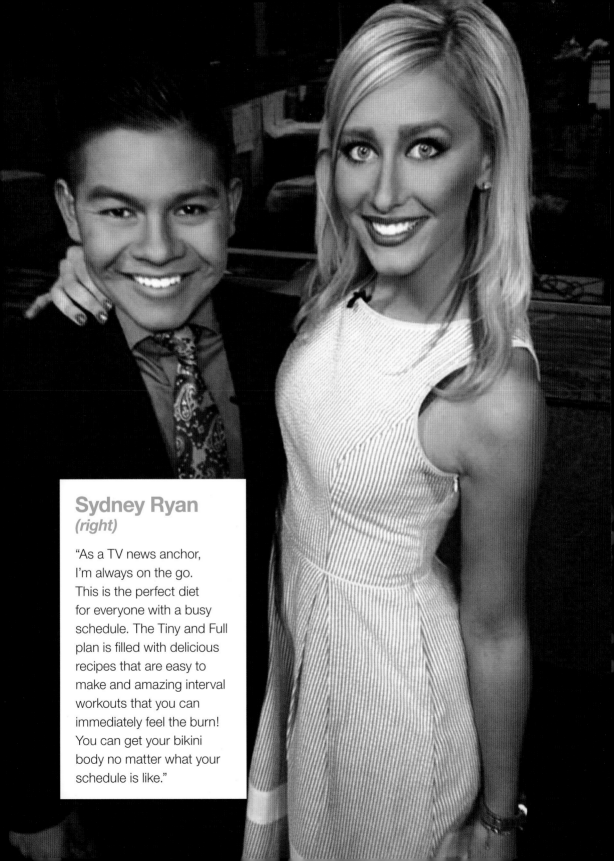

## Sydney Ryan
*(right)*

"As a TV news anchor, I'm always on the go. This is the perfect diet for everyone with a busy schedule. The Tiny and Full plan is filled with delicious recipes that are easy to make and amazing interval workouts that you can immediately feel the burn! You can get your bikini body no matter what your schedule is like."

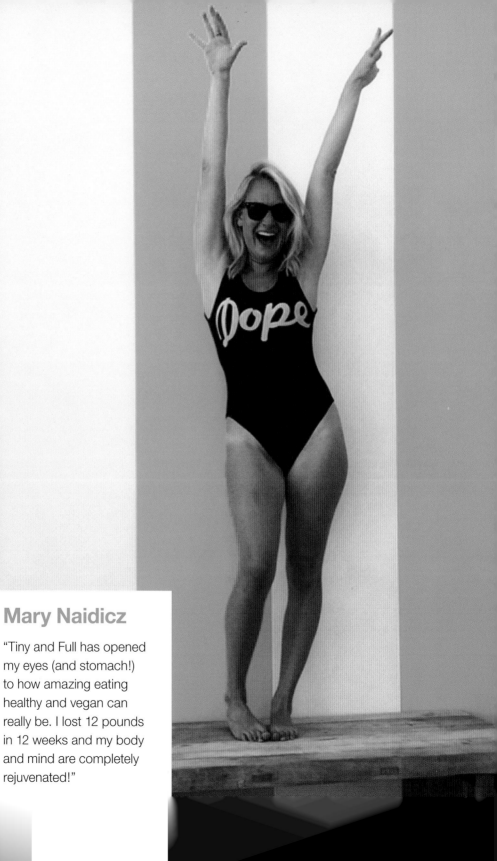

## Mary Naidicz

"Tiny and Full has opened my eyes (and stomach!) to how amazing eating healthy and vegan can really be. I lost 12 pounds in 12 weeks and my body and mind are completely rejuvenated!"

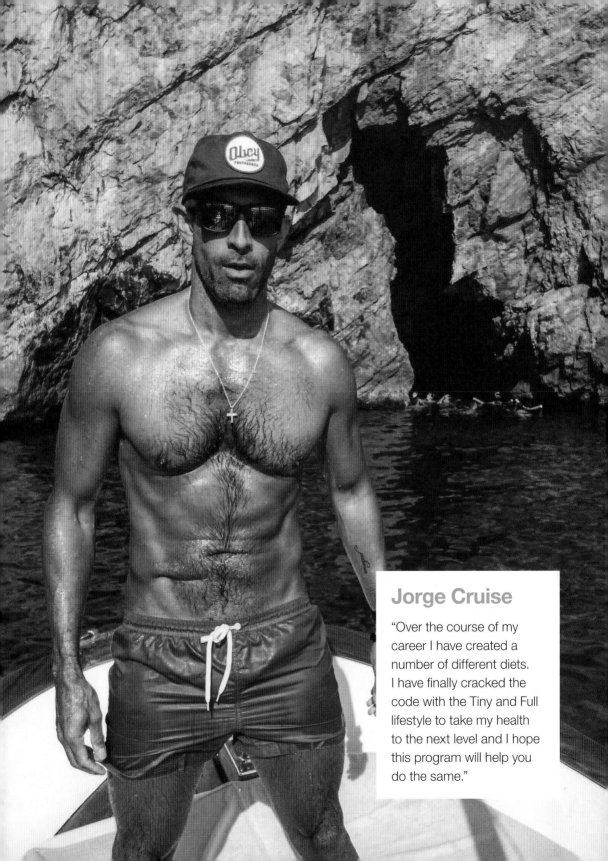

## Jorge Cruise

"Over the course of my career I have created a number of different diets. I have finally cracked the code with the Tiny and Full lifestyle to take my health to the next level and I hope this program will help you do the same."

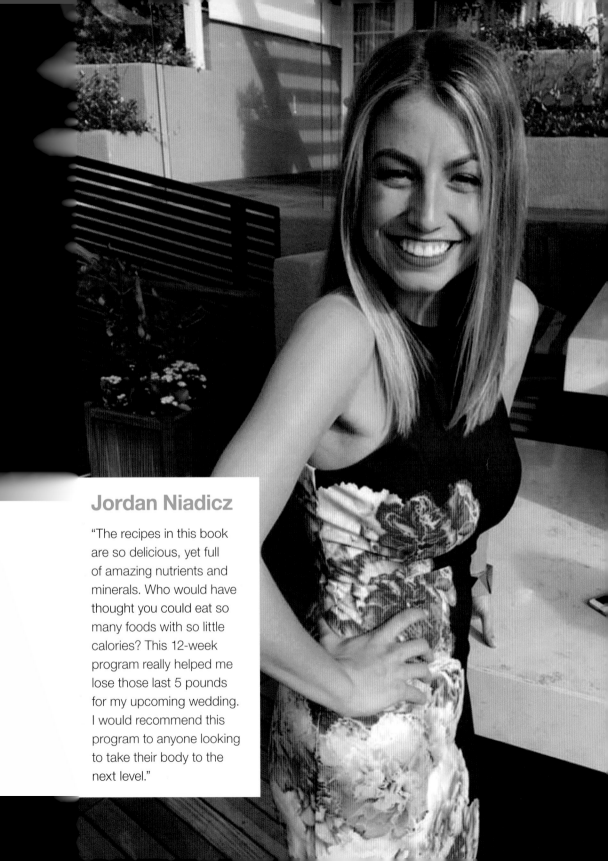

## Jordan Niadicz

"The recipes in this book are so delicious, yet full of amazing nutrients and minerals. Who would have thought you could eat so many foods with so little calories? This 12-week program really helped me lose those last 5 pounds for my upcoming wedding. I would recommend this program to anyone looking to take their body to the next level."

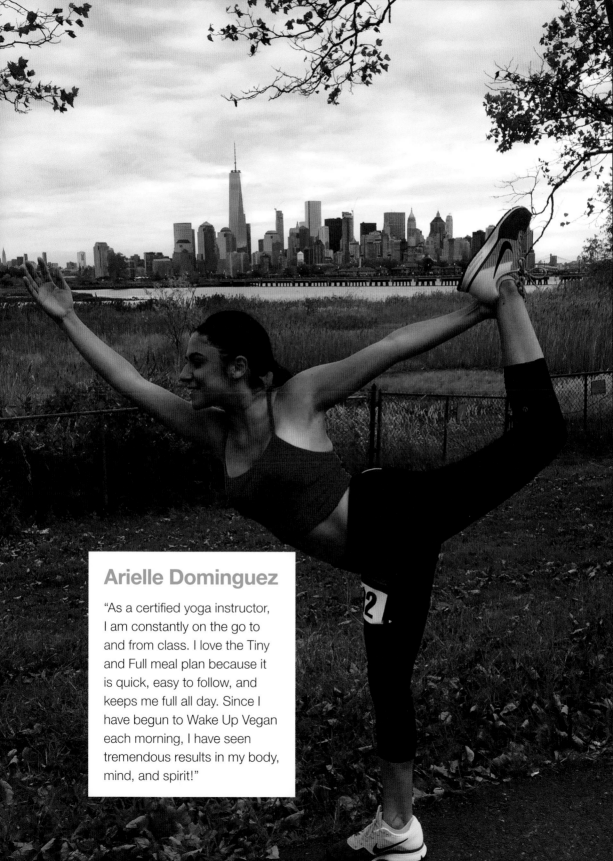

## Arielle Dominguez

"As a certified yoga instructor, I am constantly on the go to and from class. I love the Tiny and Full meal plan because it is quick, easy to follow, and keeps me full all day. Since I have begun to Wake Up Vegan each morning, I have seen tremendous results in my body, mind, and spirit!"

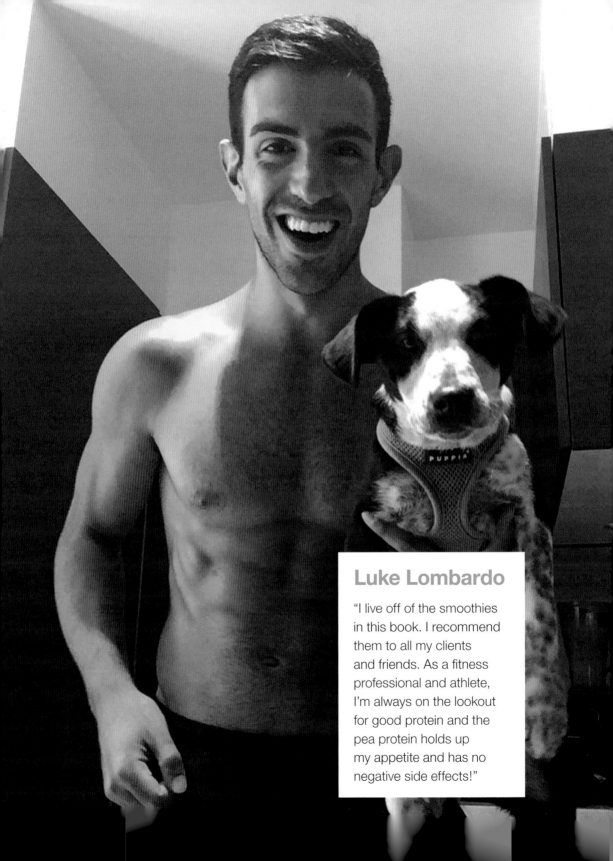

## Luke Lombardo

"I live off of the smoothies in this book. I recommend them to all my clients and friends. As a fitness professional and athlete, I'm always on the lookout for good protein and the pea protein holds up my appetite and has no negative side effects!"

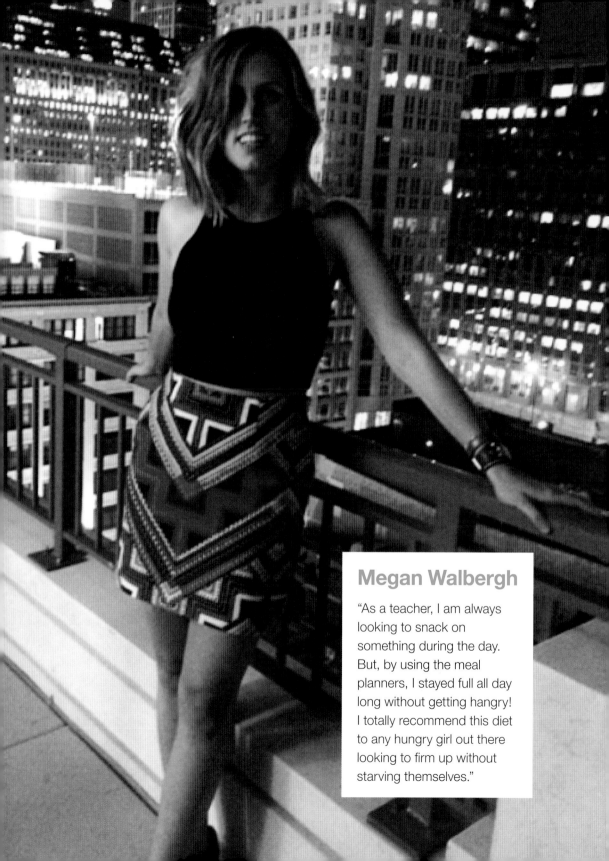

## Megan Walbergh

"As a teacher, I am always looking to snack on something during the day. But, by using the meal planners, I stayed full all day long without getting hangry! I totally recommend this diet to any hungry girl out there looking to firm up without starving themselves."

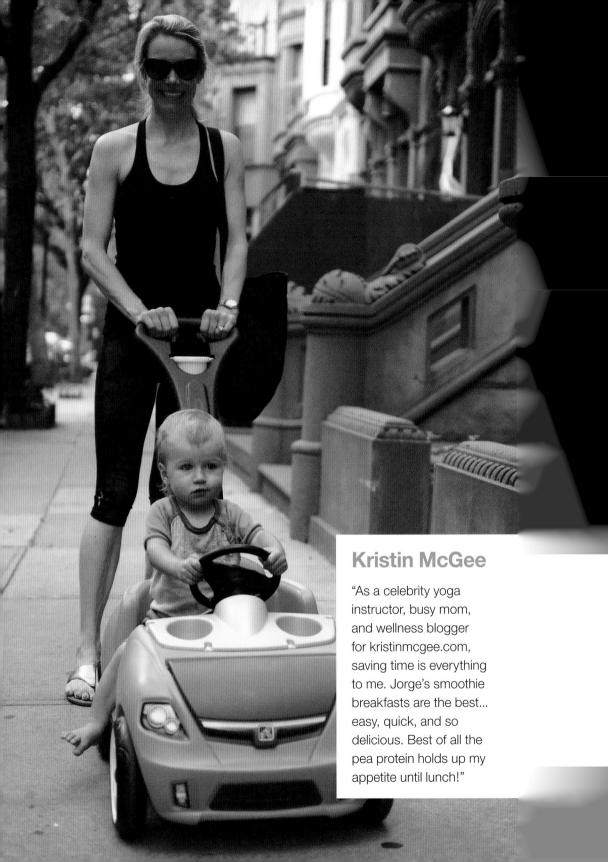

## Kristin McGee

"As a celebrity yoga instructor, busy mom, and wellness blogger for kristinmcgee.com, saving time is everything to me. Jorge's smoothie breakfasts are the best... easy, quick, and so delicious. Best of all the pea protein holds up my appetite until lunch!"

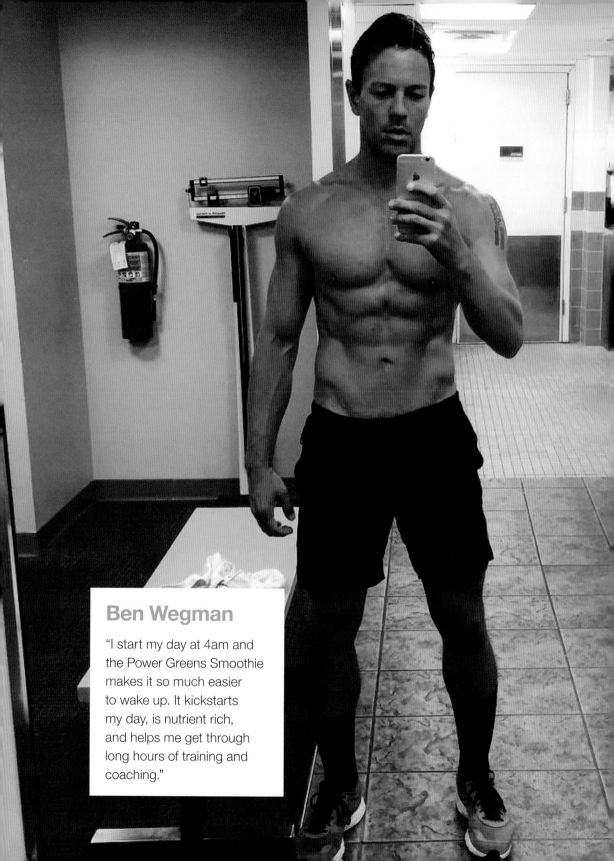

## Ben Wegman

"I start my day at 4am and the Power Greens Smoothie makes it so much easier to wake up. It kickstarts my day, is nutrient rich, and helps me get through long hours of training and coaching."

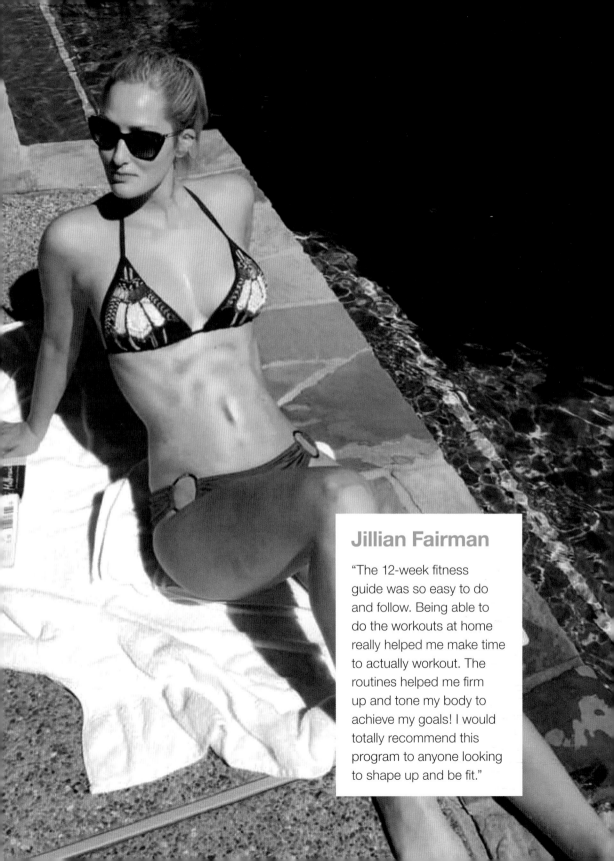

## Jillian Fairman

"The 12-week fitness guide was so easy to do and follow. Being able to do the workouts at home really helped me make time to actually workout. The routines helped me firm up and tone my body to achieve my goals! I would totally recommend this program to anyone looking to shape up and be fit."

# Selected Bibliography

## Chapter 1: Ready for Tiny

Alford, Betty, Ann Blankenship, and R. Donald Hagen. "The Effects of Variations in Carbohydrate, Protein, and Fat Content of the Diet Upon Weight Loss, Blood Values, and Nutrient Intake of Adult Obese Women." *Journal of the American Dietetic Association* 90, no. 4 (1990): 534–40.

Astrup, Arne and Søren Toubro. "Randomised Comparison of Diets for Maintaining Obese Subjects' Weight After Major Weight Loss: Ad Lib, Low Fat, High Carbohydrate Diet v Fixed Energy Intake." *British Medical Journal* 314, no. 7073 (1997): 29–34.

Bemis, Thomas, Robert Brychta, Kong Y. Chen, Amber Courville, Emma J. Crayner, Stephanie Goodwin, Juen Guo, Kevin D. Hall, Lilian Howard, Nicolas D. Knuth, Bernard V. Miller III, Carla M. Prado, Mario Siervo, Monica C. Skarulis, Mary Walter, Peter J. Walter, and Laura Yannai. "Calorie for Calorie, Dietary Fat Restriction Results in More Body Fat Loss than Carbohydrate Restriction in People with Obesity." *Cell Metabolism* 22, no. 3 (2015): 427–436.

Braun, Margaret F. and Angela Bryan. "Female Waist-to-Hip And Male Waist-to-Shoulder Ratios As Determinants Of Romantic Partner Desirability." *Journal of Social and Personal Relationships* 23, no. 5 (2006): 805–819.

Dixson, Barnaby J., Gina Grimshaw, Wayne L. Linklater, and Alan Dixson. "Watching the Hourglass." *Human Nature* 21, no. 4 (2010): 355–70.

Dixson, Barnaby J., Alan Dixson, Tim S. Jessop, Bethan J. Morgan, and Devendra Singh. "Cross-Cultural Consensus For Waist–Hip Ratio and Women's Attractiveness." *Evolution and Human Behavior* 31 (2010): 176–181.

Faries, Mark D. and John B. Bartholomew. "The Role of Body Fat in Female Attractiveness." *Evolution and Human Behavior* 15, no. 2 (2006): 672–681.

*The Devil Wears Prada.* Directed by David Frankel. Performed by Anne Hathaway, Meryl Streep. 20th Century Fox, 2006. Film.

Folsom, Aaron R., Susan A. Kaye, and Thomas A. Sellers. "Body Fat Distribution and 5-Year Risk of Death in Older Women." *The Journal of the American Medical Association* 269 (1993): 483–487.

Goetz-Perry, Catherine. "Diets With Different Targets For Intake of Fat, Protein, and Carbohydrates Achieved Similar Weight Loss in Obese Adults." *Evidence-Based Nursing* 12, no. 4 (2009): 109–109.

Hill, Kyle. "The Twinkie Diet." *Science Based Life,* November 27, 2010. <https:// sciencebasedlife.wordpress.com/2010/11/27/the-twinkie-diet/>

Hoover, Adam W., Eric R. Muth, and Jenna L. Scisco. "Examining the Utility of a Bite-Count–Based Measure of Eating Activity in Free-Living Human Beings." *Journal of the Academy of Nutrition and Dietetics* 114, no. 3 (2011): 464–469.

Jacobsen, Maryann Tomovich. "The Baby Food Diet Review: Does This Weight Loss Plan Work?" *WebMD,* December 16, 2013. <http://www.webmd.com/diet/baby-food-diet>

Just, David R. and Brian Wansink. "Trayless Cafeterias Lead Diners to Take Less Salad and Relatively More Dessert." *Public Health Nutrition* 18, no. 9 (2015): 1535–1536.

Kalm, Leah M. and Richard D. Semba. "They Starved So That Others Be Better Fed: Remembering Ancel Keys and the Minnesota Experiment." *The Journal of Nutrition* 135, no. 6 (2005): 1347–1352.

Kinsell, Laurance W., Barbara Gunning, George D. Michaels, James Richardson, Stephen E. Cox, and Calvin Lemon. "Calories Do Count." *Metabolism* 13, no. 3 (1964): 195–204.

Neporent, Liz. "Dangerous Diet Trend: The Cotton Ball Diet." *ABC News*, November 21, 2013. <http://abcnews.go.com/Health/dangerous-diet-trend-cotton-balldiet/story?id=20942888>

Nestle, Marion and Malden Nesheim. *Why Calories Count: From Science to Politics.* Oakland: University of California Press, 2013.

Nordqvist, Christian. "Nutrition Professor Loses 27 Pounds on Junk Food Diet in 10 Weeks." *Medical News Today,* November 8, 2010. <http://www.medicalnewstoday.com/articles/207071.php>

North, Jill, James E. Painter, and Brian Wansink. "Bottomless Bowls: Why Visual Cues Of Portion Size May Influence Intake." *Obesity* 13, no. 1 (2005): 93–100.

Oxford Dictionaries. "Oxford Dictionaries.com Quarterly Update: New Words Added Today Include *Hangry, Grexit,* and *Wine O'Clock*." *Oxford Dictionaries Blog*, August 27, 2015. Retrieved September 9, 2015. <http://blog.oxforddictionaries.com/press-releases/oxforddictionaries-com-quarterly-update-new-words-added-today-include-hangry-grexit-and-wine-oclock/>

Randall, Patrick K. and Devendra Singh. "Beauty Is in the Eye of the Plastic Surgeon: Waist–Hip Ratio (WHR) and Women's Attractiveness." *Personality and Individual Differences* 43, no. 2 (2007): 329–340.

Renn, Peter, Adrian Singh, and Devendra Singh. "Did the Perils of Abdominal Obesity Affect Depiction of Feminine Beauty in the Sixteenth to Eighteenth Century British Literature? Exploring the Health and Beauty Link." *Proceedings of the Royal Society B: Biological Sciences* 274, no. 1611 (2007): 891–894.

Reverby, Susan M. Review of *The Great Starvation Experiment: Ancel Keys and the Men Who Starved for Science* by Todd Tucker. *Journal of the History of Medicine and Allied Sciences* 66 (2011): 134–136.

Salis, Amanda. "The Science Behind Being 'Hangry:' Why Some People Get Grumpy When They're Hungry." *CNN*, July 20, 2015. <http://theconversation.com/health-check-the-science-of-hangry-or-why-some-people-get-grumpy-when-theyre-hungry-37229>

Singh, Devendra. "Adaptive Significance of Female Physical Attractiveness: Role of Waist-to-Hip Ratio." *Journal of Personality and Social Psychology* 65, no. 2 (1993): 293–307.

———. "Female Mate Value at a Glance: Relationship of Waist-to-Hip Ratio to Health, Fecundity and Attractiveness." *Neuroendocrinology Letters* 23, no. 4 (2002): 81–91.

———. "Female Judgment of Male Attractiveness and Desirability for Relationships: Role of Waist-to-Hip Ratio and Financial Status." *Journal of Personality and Social Psychology* 69, no. 6 (1995): 1089–1101.

———. "Mating Strategies of Young Women: Role of Physical Attractiveness." *Journal of Sex Research* 41, no. 1 (2004): 43–54.

Singh, Devendra and Dorian Singh. "Shape and Significance of Feminine Beauty: An Evolutionary Perspective." *Sex Roles* 64, no. 9 (2011): 723–731.

Singh, Devendra and Suwardi Luis. "Ethnic and Gender Consensus for the Effect of Waist-to-Hip Ratio on Judgment of Women's Attractiveness." *Human Nature* 6, no. 1 (1995): 51–65.

van Ittersum, Koert and Brian Wansink. "Portion Size Me: Plate-Size Induced Consumption Norms and Win-Win Solutions for Reducing Food Intake and Waste." *Journal of Experimental Psychology: Applied* 19, no. 4 (2013): 320–332.

Agnoli, Claudia, Benedetta Bendinelli, Carmela Calonico, Paolo Chiodini, Graziella Frasca, Sara Grioni, Giovanna Masala, Amalia Mattiello, Domenico Palli, Salvatore Panico, Carlotta Sacerdote, Calogero Saieva, Simonetta Salvini, Rosario Tumino, and Paolo Vineis. "Fruit, Vegetables, and Olive Oil and Risk of Coronary Heart Disease in Italian Women: The EPICOR Study." *American Journal of Clinical Nutrition* 93, no. 2 (2011): 275–283.

Alfredo, Martinez, Maira Bes-Rastrollo, Carmen de la Fuente Arrillaga, Miguel Ángel Martinez-González, and Almudena Sánchez-Villegas. "Association of Fiber Intake and Fruit/Vegetable Consumption with Weight Gain in a Mediterranean Population." *Nutrition* 22, no. 5 (2006): 504–511.

Alonso, Alvaro, J. Benuza, Enrique Gómez-Garcia, Miguel Ángel Martinez-González, J. Nuñez-Cordoba, and S. Palma. "Role of Vegetables and Fruits in Mediterranean Diets to Prevent Hypertension." *European Journal of Clinical Nutrition* 63, no. 5 (2008): 605–612.

Amouyel, Philippe, Jean Dallongeville, Luc Dauchet, and Serge Hercberg. "Fruit and Vegetable Consumption and Risk of Coronary Heart Disease: A Meta-Analysis of Cohort Studies." *The Journal of Nutrition* 136, no. 10 (2006): 2588–2593.

Amutha, S., S. Arulmozhiselvan, G. Hemalatha, and S. Mathanghi. "Impact of Fruit and Vegetable Intake by Healthy Subjects on the Risk Factors of Cardiovascular Diseases." *The Indian Journal of Nutrition and Dietetics* 52, no. 1 (2015): 80–87.

Appel, Lawrence J., Louise M. Bishop, Hannia Campos, Vincent J. Carey, Jeanne Charleston, Paul R. Conlin, Thomas P. Erlinger, Jeremy D. Furtado, Nancy Laranjo, Phyllis McCarron, Edgar R. Miller, Eva Obarzanek, Bernard A. Rosner, Frank M. Sacks, Janis F. Swain. "Effects of Protein, Monounsaturated Fat, and Carbohydrate Intake on Blood Pressure and Serum Lipids: Results of the OmniHeart Randomized Trial." *The Journal of the American Medical Association* 294, no. 19 (2005): 2455–2464.

Appel, Lawrence J., George A. Bray, Jeffrey A. Cutler, Marguerite A. Evans, David W. Harsha, Njeri Karanja, Pao-Hwa Lin, Marjorie McCullough, Edgar R. Miller, Thomas J. Moore, Eva Obarzanek, Frank M. Sacks, Denise Simons- Morton, Priscilla Steele, Laura P. Svetkey, Janis Swain, Thomas M. Vogt, William M. Vollmer, and Marlene M. Windhauser. "A Clinical Trial of the Effects of Dietary Patterns on Blood Pressure." *The New England Journal of Medicine* 336, no. 16 (1997): 1117–1124.

Appel, Lawrence J., Jamy D. Ard, Catherine Champagne, Njeri Karanja, Jenny H. Ledikwe, Pao-Hwa Lin, Diane C. Mitchell, Barbara J. Rolls, Helen Smiciklas- Wright, and Victor J Stevens. "Reductions in Dietary Energy Density are Associated with Weight Loss in Overweight and Obese Participants in the PREMIER Trial." *American Journal of Clinical Nutrition* 85, no. 5 (2007): 1212–1221.

Asensio, Laura, Adela Castelló, Manoli Garcia de la Hera, Jesus Vioque, and Tanja Weinbrenner. "Intake of Fruits and Vegetables in Relation to 10-Year Weight Gain Among Spanish Adults." *Obesity* 16, no. 3 (2008): 664–670.

Aucott, Lorna, Alison J. Black, William D. Fraser, Garry Duthie, Susan Duthie, Antonia C. Hardcastle, Susan A. Lanham, Helen M. Macdonald, David M. Reid, and Rena Sandison. "Effect of Potassium Citrate Supplementation or Increased Fruit and Vegetable Intake on Bone Metabolism in Healthy Postmenopausal Women: A Randomized Controlled Trial." *American Journal of Clinical Nutrition* 88, no. 2 (2008): 465–474.

Ayres, Ed. "Will We Still Eat Meat: Maybe Not, If We Wake Up to What the Mass Production of Animal Flesh is Doing to Our Health—and the Planet's." *Time*, November 8, 1999.

Barnard, Neal D., Yoshihiro Miyamoto, Kunihiro Nishimura, Tomonori Okamura, Akira Sekikawa, Misa Takegami, Makoto Wantanabe, and Yoko Yokoyama. "Vegetarian Diets and Blood Pressure." *JAMA Internal Medicine* 174, no. 4 (2014): 577–587.

Basu, Samar, Erica M. Holt, Ching Ping Hong, Antoinette Moran, Julie A. Ross, Alan R. Sinaiko, Lyn M. Steffen, and Julia Steinberger. "Fruit and Vegetable Consumption and Its Relation to Markers of Inflammation and Oxidative Stress in Adolescents." *Journal of the American Dietetic Association* 109, no. 3 (2009): 414–421.

Bazzano, Lydia A., Frank B. Hu, Kamudi Joshipura, and Tricia Y. Li. "Intake Of Fruit, Vegetables, And Fruit Juices and Risk of Diabetes in Women." *Diabetes Care* 31, no. 7 (2008): 1311–1317.

Beach, Amanda M., Julia A. Ello-Martin, Jenny H. Ledikwe, Liane S. Roe, and Barbara J. Rolls. "Dietary Energy Density in the Treatment of Obesity: A Year-Long Trial Comparing 2 Weight-Loss Diets." *American Journal of Clinical Nutrition* 85, no. 6 (2007): 1465–1477.

Bell, Elizabeth, Liane S. Roe, and Barbara Jean Rolls. "Sensory-Specific Satiety Is Affected More By Volume Than by Energy Content of a Liquid Food." *Physiology and Behavior* 78, no. 4 (2003): 593–600.

Bes-Rastrollo, Maira, Frank B. Hu, Tricia Y. Li, Miguel Ángel Martinez-González, Laura L. Sampson, and Rob M. van Dam. "Prospective Study of Dietary Energy Density and Weight Gain in Women." *The American Journal of Clinical Nutrition* 88, no. 3 (2008): 769–777.

Blanck, Heidi M., Laura Kettel Khan, Jenny H. Ledikwe, Barbara J. Rolls, Mary K. Serdula, and Jennifer D. Seymour. "Dietary Energy Density Is Associated with Energy Intake and Weight Status in US Adults." *American Journal of Clinical Nutrition* 83, no. 6 (2006): 1362–1368.

Blundell, John, Vicky Drapeau, Eric Doucet, Marion Hetherington, Neil King, and Angelo Tremblay. "Appetite Sensations and Satiety Quotient: Predictors of Energy Intake and Weight Loss." *Appetite* 48, no. 2 (2007): 159–166.

Borenstein, Amy R., Qi Dai, James C. Jackson, Eric B. Larson, and Yougui Wu. "Fruit and Vegetable Juices and Alzheimer's Disease: The Kame Project." *The American Journal of Medicine* 119, no. 9 (2006): 751–759.

Brown, Lisa, Lisa Chasan-Taber, Edward L. Giovannucci, Susan E. Hankinson, Johanna M. Seddon, Donna Spiegelman, and Walter C. Willett. "A Prospective Study of Carotenoid Intake and Risk of Cataract Extraction in US Men." *The American Journal of Clinical Nutrition* 70, no. 4 (1999): 517–524.

Buijsse, Brian, Heiner Boeing, Huaidong Du, Edith Feskens, Nita G. Forouhi, Jytte Halkjaer, Marianne U. Jakobsen, Kim Overvad, Domenico Palli, Matthias B. Schulze, Stephen Sharp, Thorkild Sørensen, Anne Tjønneland, Gianluca Tognon, Daphne L. van der A, and Nicholas J. Wareham. "Fruit and Vegetable Intakes and Subsequent Changes in Body Weight in European Populations: Results from The Project on Diet, Obesity, and Genes (DiOGenes)." *American Journal of Clinical Nutrition* 90, no. 1 (2009): 202–209.

Buring, Julia, William G. Christen, Simin Liu, and Debra A. Schaumberg. "Fruit and Vegetable Intake and the Risk of Cataract in Women." *American Journal of Clinical Nutrition* 81, no. 6 (2005): 1417–1422.

Camilleri, Michael and Anthony Lembo. "Chronic Constipation." *New England Journal of Medicine* 349 (2003): 1360–1368.

Castellanos, Vanessa, Jason C.G. Halford, Arun Kilara, D. Panyam, C.L. Pelkman, and Barbara J. Rolls. "Volume of Food Consumed Affects Satiety in Men." *American Journal of Clinical Nutrition* 67, no. 6 (1998): 1170–1177.

Centers for Disease Control and Prevention. "Low-Energy-Dense Foods and Weight Management: Cutting Calories While Controlling Hunger." <http://www.cdc.gov/nccdphp/dnpa/nutrition/pdf/r2p_energy_density.pdf>

Chiang, Yi-Chen, Zhi-Hong Jian, Pei-Chieh Ko, Chia-Chi Lung, and Oswald Ndi Nfor. "Vegetarian Diet and Cholesterol and TAG Levels by Gender." *Public Health Nutrition* 18, no. 4 (2014): 721–726.

Chylack, Leo T., Susan E. Hankinson, Paul F. Jacques, Marjorie L. McCullough, Suzen M. Moeller, Allen Taylor, Katherine L. Tucker, and Walter C. Willett. "Overall Adherence to the Dietary Guidelines for Americans Is Associated with Reduced Prevalence of Early Age-Related Nuclear Lens Opacities in Women." *Journal of Nutrition* 134, no. 7 (2004): 1812–1819.

Cole, Greg, Elizabeth Head, Donald Ingram, and James Joseph. "Nutrition, Brain Aging, and Neurodegeneration." *Journal of Neuroscience* 29, no. 41 (2009): 12795–12801.

Colditz, Graham, Frank B. Hu, Hsin-Chia Hung, Kaumudi J. Joshipura, Tricia Y. Li, Eric B. Rimm, Meir J. Stampfer, Walter C. Willett. "Intakes of Fruits, Vegetables and Carbohydrate and the Risk of CVD." *Public Health Nutrition* 12, no. 1 (2009): 115–121.

Colditz, Graham A., Frank B. Hu, Hsin-Chia Hung, David Hunter, Rui Jiang, Kaumudi J. Joshipura, Bernard Rosner, Stephanie A. Smith-Warner, Donna Spiegelman, and Walter C. Willett. "Fruit And Vegetable Intake and Risk of Major Chronic Disease." *Journal of the National Cancer Institute* 96, no. 21 (2004): 1577–1584.

De Biase, Simone Grigoletto, João Luiz Garcia Duarte, Sabrina Francine Carrocha Fernandes, and Reinaldo José Gianni. "Vegetarian Diet and Cholesterol and Triglycerides Levels." *Arquivos Brasileiros de Cardiologia* 88, no. 1 (2007): 1678–4170.

Dowling, Emily C., Neal D. Freedman, Stephanie M. George, Albert Hollenbeck, Michael F. Leitzmann, Yikyung Park, Jill Reedy, Arthur Schatzkin, and Amy F. Subar. "Fruit and Vegetable Intake and Risk of Cancer: A Prospective Cohort Study." *American Journal of Clinical Nutrition* 89, no. 1 (2009): 347–353.

Ello-Martin, Julia A., Barbara J. Rolls, and Beth C. Tohill. "What Can Intervention Studies Tell Us about the Relationship between Fruit and Vegetable Consumption and Weight Management?" *Nutrition Reviews* 62, no. 1 (2004): 1–17.

Ellwood, Kathleen C., Claudine J. Kavanaugh, and Paula R. Trumbo. "The U.S. Food And Drug Administration's Evidence-Based Review For Qualified Health Claims: Tomatoes, Lycopene, and Cancer." *Journal of the National Cancer Institute* 99, no. 14 (2007): 1074–1085.

Food and Agricultural Organization of the United Nations. "FAO Urges Action to Cope With Increasing Water Scarcity." *FAO Newsroom,* March 22, 2007. <http://www.fao.org/newsroom/en/news/2007/1000520/index.Html>

———. "Livestock a Major Threat to Environment." *FAO Newsroom,* November 29, 2006. <http://www.fao.org/newsroom/en/news/2006/1000448/index.html>

Farmer, Bonnie. "Nutritional Adequacy of Plant-Based Diets for Weight Management: Observations from the NHANES." *American Journal of Clinical Nutrition* 100, no. 1 (2014): 365S–368S.

Giovannucci, Edward, Yan Liu, Elizabeth A. Platz, Meir J. Stampfer, and Walter C. Willett. "Risk Factors for Prostate Cancer Incidence and Progression in the Health Professionals Follow-Up Study." *International Journal of Cancer* 121, no. 7 (2008): 1571–1578.

Grubard, Barry I., Richard B. Hayes, Amy E. Millen, Ulrike Peters, Amy F. Subar, Joel L. Weissfeld, Lance A. Yokochi, and Regina G. Ziegler. "Fruit and Vegetable Intake and Prevalence of Colorectal Adenoma in a Cancer Screening Trial." *American Journal of Clinical Nutrition* 86, no. 6 (2007): 1754–1764.

He, Feng J., M. Lucas, Graham A. MacGregor, and Caryl A. Nowson. "Increased Consumption of Fruit and Vegetables Is Related to a Reduced Risk of Coronary Heart Disease: Meta-analysis of Cohort Studies." *Journal of Human Hypertension* 21, no. 9 (2007): 717–728.

He, Feng J., Graham A. MacGregor, and Caryl A. Nowson. "Fruit And Vegetable Consumption and Stroke: Meta-analysis of Cohort Studies." *The Lancet* 28, no. 367 (2006): 320–326.

Kant, Ashima and B.I. Graubard. "Energy Density of Diets Reported by American Adults: Association with Food Group Intake, Nutrient Intake, and Body Weight." *International Journal of Obesity* 29, vol. 8 (2005): 950–956.

Lopes, Carla, A. Oliveira, and F. Rodríguez-Artalejo. "The Association of Fruits, Vegetables, Antioxidant Vitamins, and Fiber Intake with High-Sensitivity C- Reactive Protein: Sex and Body Mass Index Interactions." *European Journal of Clinical Nutrition* 63, no. 11 (2009): 1345–1352.

Marsh, Kate, Angela Sanders, and Carol Zeuschner. "Health Implications of a Vegetarian Diet: A Review." *American Journal of Lifestyle Medicine* 6, no. 3 (2012): 250–267.

Meengs, Jennifer S., Liane S. Roe, and Barbara J. Rolls. "Salad and Satiety: Energy Density and Portion Size of a First-Course Salad Affect Energy Intake at Lunch." *Journal of the American Dietetic Association* 104, no. 10 (2004): 1570-1576.

Messina, Ginny. "Why Do Some People Fail at Being Vegan?" *The Vegan R.D,* January 6, 2015. <http://www.theveganrd.com/2015/01/why-do-some-people-fail-at-being- vegan.html>

Natural Resources Defense Council. "Facts About Pollution from Livestock Farms." February 21, 2013. <http://www.nrdc.org/water/pollution/ffarms.asp>

Mohr, Noam. "A New Global Warming Strategy How Environmentalists are Overlooking Vegetarianism as the Most Effective Tool Against Climate Change in Our Lifetimes." *EarthSave International,* August 1, 2005. <http://www.earthsave.org/news/earthsave _global_warming_report.pdf>

Penning De Vries, F., Van Keulen, H., and Rabbinge, R. "Natural Resources and Limits of Food Production in 2040." *Systems Approaches for Sustainable Agricultural Development: Eco-Regional Approaches for Sustainable Land Use and Food Production,* edited by J. Bouma, B.A.M. Bourman, A. Kuyvenhoven, J.C. Luyten, and H.G. Zandstra, 65–87. Springer, 1995.

Petrović, Bronislav, Dragana Nikić, and Maja Nikolić. "Fruit and Vegetable Intake and the Risk for Developing Coronary Heart Disease." *Central European Journal of Public Health* 16, no. 1 (2008): 17–20.

Rolls, Barbara J. (2009). The Relationship Between Dietary Energy Density and Energy Intake." *Physiology and Behavior* 97, no. 5 (2009): 609–615.

———. *Ultimate Volumetrics Diet: Smart, Simple, Science-Based Strategies for Losing Weight and Keeping It Off.* New York: William Morrow Cookbooks, 2013.

The United Nations. "Rearing Cattle Produces More Greenhouse Gases than Driving Cars, UN Report Warns." *UN News Centre,* November 29, 2006. <http://www.un.org/apps/news/story .asp?NewsID=20772&Cr=global&Cr1=environ ment>

Wiseman, Martin. "The Second World Cancer Research Fund/American Institute for Cancer Research Expert Report. Food, Nutrition, Physical Activity, and the Prevention of Cancer: A Global Perspective." *Proceedings of the Nutrition Society* 67, no. 3 (2008): 253–256.

## Chapter 3: Ready to Wake Up

Abou-Samra, Rania, Dino Brienza, Lian Keersmaekers, Katherine Mace, Rajat Mukherjee. "Effect of Different Protein Sources on Satiation and Short-Term Satiety When Consumed as a Starter." *Nutrition Journal* 10, no. 139 (2011): 139–139.

Baumeister, Roy F. and Matthew T. Gailliot. "The Physiology Of Willpower: Linking Blood Glucose to Self-Control." *Personality and Social Psychology Review* 11, no. 4 (2007): 303–327.

Baumeister, Roy F., Matthew Gaillot, C. Nathan DeWall, and Megan Oaten. "Self-Regulation and Personality: How Interventions Increase Regulatory Success, and How Depletion Moderates the Effects of Traits on Behavior." *Journal of Personality* 74, no. 6 (2006): 1773–1802.

Baumeister, Roy F. and Andrew Vonasch. "Uses of Self-Regulation to Facilitate and Restrain Addictive Behavior." *Addictive Behaviors* 44 (2015): 3–8.

Baumeister, Roy F. and John Tierney. *Willpower: Rediscovering the Greatest Human Strength.* New York: Penguin Press, 2011.

Bell, Elizabeth A., Barbara J. Rolls, and Michelle L. Thorwart. "Water Incorporated into a Food but Not Served with a Food Decreases Energy Intake in Lean Women." *American Journal of Clinical Nutrition* 70, no. 4 (1999): 448–455.

Blundell, John, Eric Doucet, Vicky Drapeau, Marion Hetherington, Neil King, and Angelo Tremblay. "Appetite Sensations and Satiety Quotient: Predictors of Energy Intake and Weight Loss." *Appetite* 48, no. 2 (2007): 159–166.

Butryn, Meghan, James O. Hill, Suzanne Phelan, and Rena R. Wing. "Consistent Self-Monitoring of Weight: A Key Component of Successful Weight Loss Maintenance." *Obesity* 15, no. 12 (2007): 3091–3096.

Centers for Disease Control and Prevention. "Assessing Your Weight." May 15, 2015. <http://www.cdc.gov/healthyweight/assessing/index.html>

Cho, Susan, Ock Kyoung Chun, Chin Eun Chung, Saori Obayashi, and Won O. Song. "Is Consumption of Breakfast Associated with Body Mass Index in US Adults?" *Journal of the American Dietetic Association* 105, no. 9 (2005): 1373–1382.

Cho, Susan, Carol O'Neil, Theresa A. Nicklas, and Michael Zanovec. "Whole Grain and Fiber Consumption Are Associated with Lower Body Weight Measures in US Adults: National Health and Nutrition Examination Survey 1999–2004." *Nutrition Research* 30, no. 12 (2010): 815–822.

De Silva, Akila, Waljit S. Dhillo, Paul M. Matthews, and Victoria Salem. "The Use of Functional MRI to Study Appetite Control in the CNS." *Journal of Diabetes Research* (2012).

Diepvens, K., D. Häberer, and M. Westerterp-Plantenga "Different Proteins and Biopeptides Differently Affect Satiety and Anorexigenic/Orexigenic Hormones in Healthy Humans." *International Journal of Obesity* 32, no. 3 (2007): 510–518.

Foster, Gary D. and Cathy A. Nonas. "Setting Achievable Goals for Weight Loss." *Journal of the American Dietetic Association* 105, no. 5 (2005): 118–123.

Flood, Julie E. and Barbara J. Rolls. "Soup Preloads in a Variety of Forms Reduce Meal Energy Intake." *Appetite* 49, no. 3 (2007): 626–634.

Flood-Obbagy, Julie and Barbara J. Rolls. "The Effect of Fruit in Different Forms on Energy Intake and Satiety at a Meal." *Appetite* 52, no. 2 (2009): 416–422.

Goldstone, Tony. "Good Breakfast and Good Diet: New Findings Support Common Sense." Lecture presented at Neuroscience 2012, the Annual Meeting of the Society for Neuroscience, New Orleans, October 13–17, 2012.

Hill, James O., Gary K. Grunwald, Mary L. Klem, Cecilia L. Mosca, Rena R. Wing, and Holly R. Wyatt. "Long-Term Weight Loss and Breakfast in Subjects in the National Weight Control Registry." *Obesity* 10, no. 2 (2002): 78–82.

Meengs, Jennifer S., Liane S. Roe, and Barbara J. Rolls. "Salad and Satiety: Energy Density and Portion Size of a First-Course Salad Affect Energy Intake at Lunch." *Journal of the American Dietetic Association* 104, no. 10 (2004), 1570–1576.

Roe, Liane S., Barbara J. Rolls, and Rachel A. Williams. "Assessment of Satiety Depends on the Energy Density and Portion Size of the Test Meal." *Obesity* 22, no. 2 (2013): 318–324.

## Chapter 5: Your 12-Week Fitness Guide

Alméras, Natalie, Jolanda Boer, Jean-Pierre Després, E.K. Kranenbarg, and A. Tremblay. "Diet Composition and Postexercise Energy Balance." *American Journal of Clinical Nutrition* 59, no. 5 (1994): 975–979.

Alméras, Natalie, Eric Doucet, Pascal Imbeault, and Angelo Tremblay. "Physical Activity and Low-Fat Diet: Is it Enough to Maintain Weight Stability in the Reduced-Obese Individual Following Weight Loss Drug Therapy and Energy Restriction?" *Obesity Reviews* 7 (1999): 323–333.

Alméras, Natalie, Eric Doucet, A. Labrie, Denis Richard, Sylvie St-Pierre, and Mayumi Yoshioko. "Impact of High-Intensity Exercise on Energy Expenditure, Lipid Oxidation, and Body Fatness." *International Journal of Obesity* 25, no. 3 (2001): 332–339.

Bahr, Roald and O.M. Sejersted. "Effect of Intensity of Exercise on Excess Postexercise O2 Consumption." *Metabolism* 40, no. 8 (1991): 836–841.

Bielinski, R., Yves Schutz, and E. Jéquier. "Energy Metabolism During the Postexercise Recovery in Man." *The American Journal of Clinical Nutrition* 42, no. 1 (1985): 69–82.

Bonen, Arend, Stuart D.R. Galloway, George J.F. Heigenhauser, Lawrence L. Spriet, and Jason L. Talanian. "Two Weeks of High-Intensity Aerobic Interval Training Increases the Capacity for Fat Oxidation During Exercise in Women." *Journal of Applied Physiology* 102, no. 4 (2007): 1439–1447.

Bonen, Arend, George J.F. Heigenhauser, Christopher G.R. Perry, and Lawrence L. Spriet. "High-Intensity Aerobic Interval Training Increases Fat and Carbohydrate Metabolic Capacities in Human Skeletal Muscle. *Applied Physiology, Nutrition, and Metabolism* 33, no. 6 (2008): 1112–1123.

Bouchard, Claude, Jean-Aimé Simoneau, and Angelo Tremblay. "Impact of Exercise Intensity on Body Fatness and Skeletal Muscle Metabolism." *Metabolism* 43, no. 7 (1994): 814–818.

Boutcher, Steve. "High-Intensity Intermittent Exercise and Fat Loss." *Journal of Obesity* (2011).

Boutcher, Steve, D.J. Chisholm, Judith Fruend, and Ethlyn Gail Trapp. "The Effects of High-Intensity Intermittent Exercise Training on Fat Loss and Fasting Insulin Levels of Young Women." *International Journal of Obesity* 32, no. 4 (2008): 684–691.

Cloud, John. "Why Exercise Won't Make You Thin." *Time,* August 9, 2009. <http://content .time.com/time/printout/0,8816,1914974,00.html>

Cohn, V. "Passion to Keep Fit: 100 Million Americans Exercising." *Washington Post,* August 31, 1980.

Craig, C.L., Jean-Pierre Després, Blake Ferris, C. Leblanc, Torrance T. Stephens, and Angelo Tremblay. "Effect of Intensity of Physical Activity on Body Fatness and Fat Distribution." *The American Journal of Clinical Nutrition* 51, no. 2 (1990): 153–157.

Dawes, Jay and Brad Schoenfeld. "High-Intensity Interval Training: Applications for General Fitness Training." *Strength and Conditioning Journal* 31, no. 6 (2009): 44–46.

Dionne, Isabell, M. Johnson, Sylvie St-Pierre, Angelo Tremblay, and Matthew White. "Acute Effect of Exercise and Low-Fat Diet on Energy Balance in Heavy Men." *International Journal of Obesity and Related Metabolic Disorders* 21, no. 5 (1997): 413–416.

Ebbeling, Cara B., Henry A. Feldman, Erica Garcia-Lago, David L. Hachey, David S. Ludwig, Janis F. Swain, and William W. Wong. "Dietary Composition on Energy Expenditure During Weight-Loss Maintenance." *Journal of the American Medical Association* 307, no. 24 (2012): 2627–2634.

Fissinger, Jean A., Christopher L. Melby, and Darlene A. Sedlock. "Effect of Exercise Intensity and Duration on Postexercise Energy Expenditure." *Medicine and Science in Sports Exercise* 21, no. 6 (1989): 662–666.

Fogelholm, Mikael and K. Kukkonen-Harjula. "Does Physical Activity Prevent Weight Gain: A Systematic Review." *Obesity Reviews* 1, no. 2 (2000): 95–111.

Hirsch, Jules, Rudolph L. Leibel, and Michael Rosenbaum. "Energy Expenditure Resulting from Altered Body Weight." *New England Journal of Medicine* 332, no. 10 (1995): 621–628.

Hamilton E.J., D.M. Koceja, and W.C. Miller. "A Meta-Analysis of the Past 25 Years of Weight Loss Research Using Diet, Exercise, or Diet Plus Exercise Intervention." *International Journal of Obesity* 21, no. 10 (1997): 941–947.

Jenkins, David G. and Paul Laursen. "The Scientific Basis for High-Intensity Interval Training: Optimising Training Programmes and Maximising Performance in Highly Trained Endurance Athletes." *Sports Medicine* 32, no. 1 (2002): 53–73.

McBride, Jeffery M., Richard P. Mikat, and Mark D. Schuenke. "Effect of an Acute Period of Resistance Exercise on Excess Post-Exercise Oxygen Consumption: Implications for Body Mass Management." *European Journal of Applied Physiology* 86, no. 5 (2002): 411–417.

Schoenfeld, Brad. "Does Cardio After an Overnight Fast Maximize Fat Loss?" *Strength and Conditioning Journal* 33, no. 1 (2011): 23–25.

Van Dusen, Allison. "Ten Ways to Get More From Your Workout." *Forbes,* October 20, 2008. <http://www.forbes.com/2008/10/20/exercise-workout-shorter-forbeslife- cx _avd_1020health_slide_5.html?thisSpeed=30000>

Selected Bibliography

# Acknowledgments

I owe particular gratitude to my amazing team, as without them, nothing would be possible. To Kristin Penne, for keeping us all organized, on time, and sane. And for all of the wonderful work you did on creating menus, recipes, and other priceless research. To Oliver Stephenson, I could not have done this project without your direction and support. You truly know how to apply your incredible commitment and talent to our mission. You make it all run! Thank you for your invaluable research and insights. And to Marianne McGinnis, for helping me express my thoughts to the world. Without the hard work from each of you, this book would not exist.

A big thank you to the amazing BenBella Books team: Adrienne Lang, Sarah Dombrowsky, Leah Wilson, Heather Butterfield, Monica Lowry, Jennifer Canzoneri, Rachel Phares, Alicia Kania—and, most especially, to Glenn Yeffeth, for supporting my vision of this project and helping me share it with the world. Thank you for all of your hard work and support, it means so much.

Thank you to the Perseus team as well for helping get this book out: David Steinberger, Elena Chmilowski, Jessie Borkan, Andrea Gochnauer, Sabrina McCarthy, Heidi Sachner, Kim Highland, and Maha Khalil.

A very special thank you to my fiancé, Sam Ayers. Your support with this project has been incredible. Your insights are invaluable, thank you for all that you did to help me bring this book to life. And to my two sons, Parker and Owen, thank you for being such fun, loving boys. I love watching you grow up and I love being your dad.

I'd also like to thank my friends and supporters: Richard Galanti, Barrie Galanti, Pennie Clark-Ianniciello, Ginnie Roeglin, Tim Talevich, Mary Ellen-Keathing, Edward Ash-Milby, Jon Foro, Sherman Griffin, John Redmann, Leslie Marcus, Lisa Gregorisch-Dempsey, Patty Serato, Carol Brooks, Maggie Jacqua, James Avenell, Christine Byun, Nicolette Gebhardt, Brandon Baiden, Talia Parkinson, Natalie Bubnis, Scott Eason, Patty Neger, Mario Lopez, Tim Sullivan, Dr. Mehmet Oz, Dr. David Katz, Dr. Andrew Weil, Dr. Christiane Northrup, President Bill Clinton, Senator Hillary Clinton, Jennifer Wilson, Emma Maliszewski, Jules Barker, Kate Bedrick, Gabriella Soto, Lindsey Groginski, Phil Lobel, Shaun Kimbrow, David Jackson, Jacqui Stafford, Marissa Gold, Dory Larrabee-Zayas, Nicole Friday, Lacy Looney, Bob Wietrak, Denise Vivaldo, Jonathan Lizoette, Frank Rizzo, Jessica Scosta, Tory Jacob, Nicole Blinn.

# About the Author

"Eat well without dieting or going to the gym with Jorge's strategies for breakfast, lunch, and dinner."

— Mehmet Oz, MD, host of *The Dr. Oz Show*

"Jorge Cruise gets it right. His recipes and quick options make eating smart easy. I recommend them highly."

— Andrew Weil, MD, director of the Arizona Center for Integrative Medicine, University of Arizona, and author of *Why Our Health Matters*

JORGE CRUISE is internationally recognized as a leading celebrity fitness trainer and is the #1 bestselling author of more than 20 books in 16 languages, with more than 6 million books in print. He is a contributor to *The Steve Harvey Show, The Dr. Oz Show, Extra TV, Good Morning America, The Today Show, The Rachael Ray Show,* Huffington Post, *First for Women* magazine, and the *Costco Connection.* He hosts *The Jorge Cruise Show* with more than 12 million listeners.

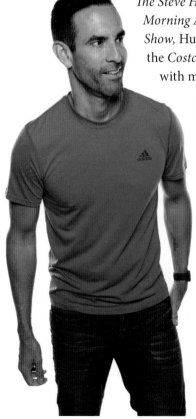

Jorge received his bachelor's degree from the University of California, San Diego (UCSD) and his fitness credentials from the Cooper Institute for Aerobics Research, the American College of Sports Medicine (ACSM), and the American Council on Exercise (ACE).

Jorge's career was launched on *The Oprah Winfrey Show* in November of 1998. From there, he was featured in *The Oprah Magazine* in the January 2005 issue and featured again in her book *O's Guide to Life.*

Celebrities who have since followed Jorge's diet plans include Angelina Jolie, Jennifer Lopez, Lucy Liu, Kyle Richards, Eva Longoria, Chrissy Teigen, and, most recently, Steve Harvey.

# Join my **FREE** Email Club
# to get a full-length
# workout video from the book

Visit tinyandfull.com/workout to join my FREE Email Club to get a full length workout video that walks you through the steps of the whole routine. Also, as a bonus you get my newest recipes with my favorite meals as well as interviews and updates to events, deals and promotions.

(Valued at $79.95)

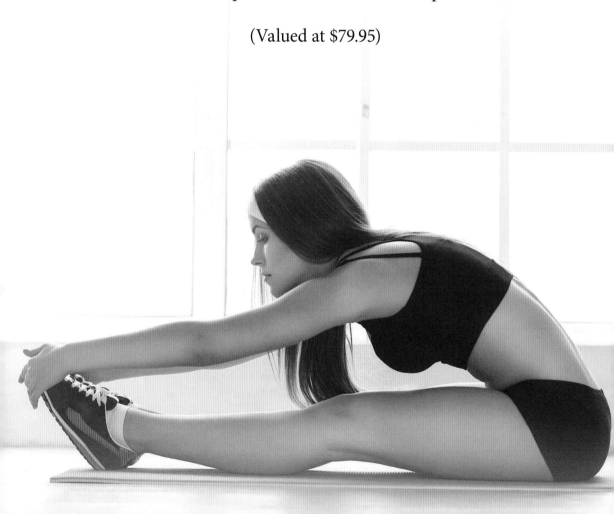